T0208984

The author lets her light for Jesus shine through in all she does. A true encourager to all! Her life mission is to share her love for the Lord with others, in hopes that they know Him by his love. Bright, uplifting, full of joy in all circumstances. **STACEY WINK**

Tumors... brain surgery... those are some very scary words to hear and even more terrifying when referring to yourself or someone you love. Jeaunetta shares her very personal journey of going through brain surgery and living to tell about it while demonstrating a walking (or sometimes stumbling) testimony of love, laughter, and what the power of putting all of your faith and trust in the Lord can do. **CARMEN CAROTHERS**

Jeaunetta doesn't just encourage others with the gospel, she lives it out. Some folks think that being a Christian means you will never have struggles, fears or doubts. But Christ never said that. He said in this world you WILL have struggles, but take heart I have overcome the world. She has overcome SO much, and has never lost heart. She has one of the biggest hearts I know of. She has been a source of encouragement for so many. Even when I know she probably wasn't feeling the best, she always has something funny or sweet to say. The light and love of Christ just flows from her. Jeaunetta is a blessing to all she meets. **WENDY MCDONNELL**

Jeaunetta has the most positive outlook on life and I am thankful to be her friend. She lives out her favorite verse in Nehemiah 8:10. She uses the Joy of the Lord to help her find the strength to encourage others. That strength comes from her close relationship with Christ. She knows he holds her hand. This is the message she shares daily with others. **DONNA HARMAN**

In addition to raising a family and being a good wife, mother and friend, Jeaunetta has always found time to get actively involved in ministering and encouraging those around her. Even in the midst of her own excruciating trials with her health, Jeaunetta remained steadfast as she always looked for an opportunity to minister and bring joy to others. I had the joy of witnessing her selflessly bring comfort and joy to brain surgery patients just days after her own surgery. Jeaunetta is a testimony of what selfless love is and I am honored to call her my friend. She is precious and her love for God and others radiates. **ANGELA HAHN**

It's seems unreal, but I've known Jeaunetta for 30 years! During these years I've witnessed her life. She has had some difficult times physically, spiritually and emotionally. When life gave her "lemons" she chose to trust the LORD and faithfully depend upon His goodness and His promises. When she shares - whether it's at the kitchen table or in a ladies conference, she has you right there with her, laughing, crying, singing... Whether it's only "brain surgery," or _____ (you fill in the blank).

Jeaunetta will point you to the loving Lord who will get you through your situation with a smile on your face, a song in your heart and a testimony to share with others. Thank you for blessing us, dear Jeaunetta! **PASTOR CONNIE MUNDT**

I MARVEL at this girl! Her smile is a mile wide even with a plate in her head and the long road of recovery from brain surgery. This is just the tip of the iceberg with Jeaunetta. She knows a scripture song for every need AND how to sing it. She's always encouraging someone else even when she is the one in need. Jeaunetta has been doing programs for children and women for years, but this time it's different: this is about trusting God when her own future hangs in the balance. Is God all those things that she's been saying He is? Is He enough to be trusted when she wants to bolt out the doors of the hospital and forget the whole business of this brain surgery? He is and more. For every fear she faced, Jesus met her there. Jeaunetta is an amazing woman of God, but she won't take any of the credit - it's all His. I'm looking forward to reading this book. I've seen her LIVE this story: it's all about walking through the fire with the JOY of the LORD - and the support of friends. (and she has many, because of the Spirit within her - God's Holy Spirit.) **LAUREL FRIEDL**

Jeaunetta brings joy and encouragement to all she meets. Even in the midst of overwhelming circumstances, Jeaunetta looks for ways to be a blessing and encouragement to others. The Joy of the Lord truly is her strength! **SANDY MCLATCHIE**

Jeaunetta has spoken at a number of ladies' events and retreats for our women's ministry. She has a positively contagious spirit about her that engages all ages to reignite or deepen their love for Christ. Jeaunetta's enthusiasm and passion can be seen in her coordination efforts to provide a program that is perfect for your needs. I highly recommend you invite Jeaunetta to speak at your next women's event, you will not regret it! **LAURI DOMER, DIRECTOR OF WOMEN'S MINISTRIES, RIVER VALLEY ALLIANCE CHURCH**

Tender love & compassion comes to life as Jeaunetta expresses God's goodness to her through adversity and trials. What a joy and blessing! She's the real deal! **ROBBIE FOSTER, MOTHER & FRIEND**

Jeaunetta's life is a living testimony of courage, strength, hope and love that she draws from God. Her story of facing adversity will encourage and inspire her readers. **CAROL ANDRLE**

You'll laugh, you'll cry... Gets to the heart of the gospel and how to live it out in the real world. Speaks from personal experience with real trials and points us to Jesus, the one who gives us JOY in whatever circumstances we find ourselves. **PASTOR DAVE & NANCY ZIMMERMAN**

DON'T PANIC,
IT'S ONLY
BRAIN
SURGERY!

MY JOURNEY FROM
PANIC to PEACE

JEAUNETTA WESTENBERG

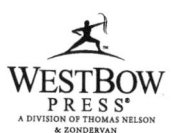

WESTBOW
PRESS®
A DIVISION OF THOMAS NELSON
& ZONDERVAN

Scripture taken from the King James Version of the Bible

Scripture quotations marked (NIV) are taken from the Holy Bible, New International Version®, NIV®. Copyright © 1973, 1978, 1984, 2011 by Biblica, Inc.™ Used by permission of Zondervan. All rights reserved worldwide. www.zondervan.com The "NIV" and "New International Version" are trademarks registered in the United States Patent and Trademark Office by Biblica, Inc.™

Scripture quotations are taken from the Holy Bible, New Living Translation, copyright ©1996, 2004, 2007, 2013, 2015 by Tyndale House Foundation. Used by permission of Tyndale House Publishers, Inc., Carol Stream, Illinois 60188. All rights reserved.

The Holy Bible, English Standard Version® (ESV®) Copyright © 2001 by Crossway, a publishing ministry of Good News Publishers. All rights reserved. ESV Text Edition: 2016

This book is a work of non-fiction. Unless otherwise noted, the author and the publisher make no explicit guarantees as to the accuracy of the information contained in this book and in some cases, names of people and places have been altered to protect their privacy.

WestBow Press books may be ordered through booksellers or by contacting:

WestBow Press
A Division of Thomas Nelson & Zondervan
1663 Liberty Drive
Bloomington, IN 47403
www.westbowpress.com
1 (866) 928-1240

Because of the dynamic nature of the Internet, any web addresses or links contained in this book may have changed since publication and may no longer be valid. The views expressed in this work are solely those of the author and do not necessarily reflect the views of the publisher, and the publisher hereby disclaims any responsibility for them.

Any people depicted in stock imagery provided by Thinkstock are models, and such images are being used for illustrative purposes only. Certain stock imagery © Thinkstock.

ISBN: 978-1-9736-0708-3 (sc)
ISBN: 978-1-9736-0709-0 (hc)
ISBN: 978-1-9736-0707-6 (e)

Library of Congress Control Number: 2017917444

Print information available on the last page.

WestBow Press rev. date: 11/29/2017

This book is dedicated to my entire family who has loved me, supported me and encouraged me! They have helped me through every stage of my life and my recovery. (Especially my Mother who has been my greatest example of living victoriously in the storm.) God has truly blessed me with wonderful parents, a sweet and faithful husband, two adorable boys, awesome and encouraging sisters (and their husbands), a kind brother (and his wife), a sweet Mother-in-Law and my husband's brother and sisters and their spouses. All of whom, I am so grateful for!

SPECIAL THANKS

I am so grateful to have a loving family and faithful friends who prayed for, encouraged, cooked for my family and cared for me on this long road from panic to peace. Thanks to their generosity, my family was taken care of (and well-fed), which was such a blessing.

- *Thank you to all of the faithful Prayer Warriors who flooded the throne on my behalf and those who continue to faithfully pray for myself and my family!*
- *Thank you to Hilary Furnish Photography for the fun and laughs during our photo shoots.*
- *Thank you to the following church families who were such a blessing throughout my situation for both myself and my family: Watertown Community Church, River Valley Alliance Church, Faith Lutheran Church, Good Shepherd Lutheran Church.*
- *Thank you to Megan Schmieder and Donna Rantanen who helped with editing and proofing.*
- *Thank you to the Butch Mayer Family for help with our home.*
- *Thank you to the Ladies that allow me to minister to them and share my many stories of God's faithfulness to their church groups.*

"Don't Panic is a very up close, personal, overwhelming and yet sometimes hysterical reflection of my personal health struggles with a brain tumor. I am still amazed at how the Lord worked on my heart and my mind to help me through brain surgery, and a very lengthy rehabilitation process. Don't Panic became a "HOW TO" book of life lessons and a Bible study for anyone going through a difficult situation. It was written through laughter and tears, as I share some very vulnerable moments in my recovery. I was blessed by the lessons I learned while claiming victory over panic and anxiety as I experienced things that were out of my control. It was in those moments that the Lord touched my life and taught me how to get through even the most overwhelming circumstances. I cannot tell you how many times I have said the following phrase to myself after my first meeting with my neurosurgeon... Don't Panic, It's Only Brain Surgery!" - Jeaunetta Westenberg

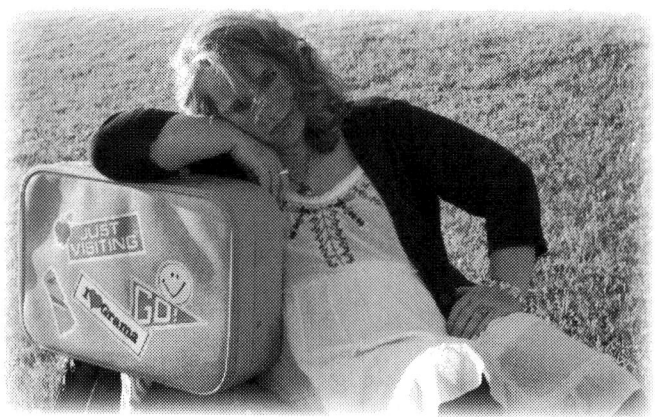

"Sometimes the hardest journeys are the ones we try to travel alone..." Jeaunetta Westenberg

CONTENTS

INTRODUCTION

I guess it's like they say; life is full of little surprises. Some are good and some are not. There are even times when we go through things that shake the very core of our being, and lead us to draw upon our faith in the Lord like never before.

When this happens, no matter how hard it is, or how hopeless we feel, we need to rest on the promise (and the fact) that GOD alone is in control of all things. That includes myself and my circumstances, even when things seemed impossible.

My story was really a tough one to tell. Things did seem impossible as I struggled through brain tumors, brain surgery, spastic quadriplegia, and a very long recovery. I learned throughout my own situation to cling to His promises, and I am blessed by this verse in Jeremiah that reminds me of the hope I have in Him for my future.

> **"For I know the plans I have for you,"** declares the LORD, **"plans to prosper you and not to harm you, plans to give you hope and a future."**
> **Jeremiah 29:11(NIV)**

That verse also reminded me that my plans are not His plans for my life. When things go wrong in this life, what a comfort it is to know that God already has a plan for us that is filled with hope for a prosperous future. Those plans, and that hope, are promised to give us something to stand on when we feel like there is sinking sand all around us. I can tell you that I have felt that sinking sand under my feet, but instead of allowing it to collapse and swallow me up, I learned (with the Lord's help) that I needed to just release everything and totally rely on Him. It has not been an easy process but the Lord has really been at work in my situation.

In this book, I want to share how God works within our circumstances, and specifically how He has worked through mine, to show me that He is there. No matter how dire things may seem, or how far we have sunk into the muck and the mire, He will offer strength and even give JOY during the hardest of times. If you are struggling with anything right now and questioning every part of your circumstances, no matter what they are, I want you to know that you are not alone and, this book has definitely been written for you.

Throughout my journey into the world of tumors and brain surgery, and all of the scary things that accompany such a difficult diagnosis, I have struggled with the devastating fear of the unknown. At times, I became overwhelmed with a panic so real, and so disabling I thought it could overtake me. I had gone through struggles with anxiety before, but never experienced panic so real and overwhelming. There were times I felt so down and defeated I thought I would never make it through the battle. I traveled a long road to recovery and it was hard. Starting with the basics, I had to relearn the simplest of tasks. It was everything that I always did so easily yet took for granted. That, in itself, was draining both physically and mentally.

After I started my intense rehab program in the hospital, I remember the therapists helping me to walk for the very first time. It was quite an overwhelming experience. I felt so defeated and my emotions really got the best of me. The tears just flowed down my face as I struggled to move, my body shaking uncontrollably with each movement. Two people helped me to stand and another would move each foot one step at a time. I felt so out of control and had to have help to keep my legs from buckling beneath me. I still recall praying and hoping that my body would stop shaking and simply remember how to comply with movements that should have been like second nature to me. The physical therapists would hold my hands to a walker in front of me and have another person follow closely behind with a wheel chair. They were there for that moment when I just couldn't go anymore. It was so hard and all I really wanted to do was give up, because it took everything out of me. I noticed with every move I made, I was struggling just to see clearly. It seemed as if the harder I tried, the blurrier everything appeared around me. I was so exhausted and I could not see the people or the hallway ahead. All of my surroundings seemed to be spinning, and it felt as if I was frozen in time. I would look all around me but all I could see was the struggle. It was so hard and totally overwhelming. Was God actually using this opportunity to teach me a most valuable life lesson? I started to wonder about that after my walk, and to think about my life… How many times has that happened to me? I am not talking about trying to walk, I am talking about not being able to see things clearly. I could not see all that was going on around me because the struggle was right there, in my line of sight, and all I could focus on. I believe that happens to all of us as we go through a difficult situation in life. The struggle is the only thing we can see, so it is nearly impossible to get past it. It is quite overwhelming.

During that first walk, I cried as I took each step, I wasn't sure if I was crying because I was hurting, or if I was sad, or if I was simply overwhelmed because of my condition? The hardest part was that I felt alone in my circumstances. I had to continually remind myself that I was never alone because God was always there beside me. He knew exactly what I was going through. He was right there with each and every step. I needed to remember that He has promised to always be there. He loves me and even cares about my struggle. I am so thankful the Bible reminds me that He even cares about all of my tears.

Psalm 56:8 (NLT) says...

> *You keep track of all my sorrows, you have collected all my tears in your bottle. You have recorded each one in your book.*

What a comfort to know that our Heavenly Father sees our circumstances and even knows our sorrows.

You may be asking at this point... Who am I and why am I sharing my story? I am sharing my story because I know that there are so many out there who are struggling and trying to get through a tough time. If any of the things I have learned can help someone else as they try to navigate through stormy waters, or struggle with an anxious heart, then I feel that the Lord has used my situation for His glory and it is worth all I have been through. I cannot tell you how comforting it was after my diagnosis, for me to hear from others who have endured similar circumstances. I want to be that comfort to someone else, as well.

Anyone who knows me knows how I love this life that the Lord has blessed me with. I love being able to share His love in the ministry, and He has filled my heart with a love for others. I want more than anything to be an encourager who shares the bright side of everything, especially in the most trying of times. I also love living fully in the Joy of the Lord and sharing funny stories about all of life's moments.

That is why I am sharing my story with each of you. I want you to know that, in spite of the pain you may be experiencing, God can and will give you a peace that passes all understanding and fill your heart with an overflowing Joy.

I have not had an easy time these past few years, and as I write it down, I start to remember some of the lowest chapters in my life that I feel I should share. It is my prayer that through this book you will be encouraged and see that there is victory in Christ Jesus no matter what you are going through.

My story is not a sad one by any means. It is very important for me to share the struggles, but even more than that, I must share the blessings. Because no matter what you are going through in your life, God can and will work it out for His glory. I want to encourage you through my story of victory, not sadness.

As I talk about these things, I am reminded of a program I heard so many years ago that really made an impact on me and my ministry.

I sat in an audience of about 1500 women who were looking to be inspired. We waited eagerly to listen to a woman who would be sharing encouragement, JOY and peace at Christmas time.

This was at a time in my life when I could really have used some encouragement and certainly needed the JOY. I could not wait to hear her advice on how we could live a better life and enjoy all of the good things that come from Christ. As the program started, the speaker shared a sad story that made everyone cry. I thought to myself as a speaker: wow, she really knows how to engage an audience. Then another horribly sad story was told, and another, and still another.

Finally, we were nearing the end of the program and I must say, I was so disappointed. I had used up all of the tissues in my bag and I must have looked like a blubbering mess. Her sad stories left me more discouraged than ever. I felt so bad for this poor woman. Surely, the program wasn't over. She had to have something more to share! Something beautiful? Something good? I really needed that happily ever after moment. After all, the program was supposed to be on joy... Where was the JOY? Where was the VICTORY?

I came to be inspired, but I was leaving empty and even more drained than when I arrived. Thinking of this experience made me more determined than ever to show all aspects of my recovery, but mostly to highlight how the Lord has brought me through it. That is the story that we need to hear and the message that we need to know. The hard truth is, God may not deliver us from our trials, but I can say for certain that He will always walk right alongside us to help us through it. God is faithful and even when there is no miracle in this life, we can rest assured that He is still God and we can still walk in victory.

Have you ever felt like I did after I saw that program? Maybe you just need to hear a success story to keep you moving forward? I am happy to say that despite my disappointments, the Lord really used that program in my life to show me that no matter what we are going through, our focus should NEVER be only on the struggle. We do need to recognize the struggle, but we need to focus on the VICTORY.

Sometimes, just like the time when I was walking with the physical therapists, our focus is skewed and we might even discover we are facing the wrong way. We need to look forward and fix our eyes on the plan that God has for us. It can be really hard, but we need to allow him to lead us through troubled times.

The purpose of this book is not to focus on my brain tumors, the surgery, or the panic I experienced; it is to show how God took me from PANIC to PEACE and how He can do the same for you. It was not an easy road, and I did not always take the right path, but I did experience victories throughout my recovery.

Sharing the victories does not mean there were no struggles. I will share those struggles and how God helped me through them. He showed me, through His Word and through others, that in the midst of any storm we can claim His peace that passes all understanding. God ALWAYS has a plan and will show us how to be resilient in any situation. It is so comforting to know His plans are perfect and His Joy is the prescription for all that ails us. I want us to remember: it doesn't matter what we are going through, we can give it to Him!

In the following chapters, I will share how I leaned on the joy of the Lord, even when I was overwhelmed with an anxious heart. In my story, I changed the way I was seeing my circumstances and told myself over and over again… DON'T Panic, It's Only Brain Surgery!

FROM PANIC TO PEACE

Life is not always easy for anyone. My life certainly has not been an exception and my story could be told by so many. For me, my greatest struggle has been that with my health. I have dealt with health troubles that have at times really hindered my quality of life. I was limited in my abilities and my health definitely affected what I wanted to do or dreamed of doing. Due to my health issues, I felt as if I had to give up so many things that I thought were important. I used to enjoy bike riding, walking, dancing and so many other activities. It was difficult to let go of the things I loved. It was hard to lose those friends who still wanted to do those things I could no longer participate in. As time went by, the season for those friendships ended. Even though my health kept me from doing some things, I tried so hard to not let it keep me from LIVING.

I needed to look at it like this… I had to adapt and maybe even change the way I did things. Sure, I would miss some of my favorite pastimes and friendships that I enjoyed, but I knew that there were other things that I could look forward to. I even tried to accept it as a challenge and look at what I was still able to do that so many can't.

I did learn that I should never be so attached to something that I cannot be happy doing something else. Sometimes change is hard, but I have learned that it can also be a blessing.

Throughout my life, and these challenges, through the tears and the pain, I tried to look at the silver lining. I believed that I had a very firm foundation when it came to my emotional well-being and considered myself a very laid-back and peaceful personality. I was not someone who usually flew off the handle or overreacted to anything. I really thought I could just roll with the punches, even during the past few years dealing with the scary process of brain surgery.

I did not think that I would let anything shake me, but I noticed that my laid-back personality started taking a back seat to a rush of emotional and fearful thoughts as the reality of my circumstances started to weigh on my mind.

I must say, it really surprised me how panic came over me so slowly that I did not even recognize it. It was stealing my peace, and thereby breaking up my foundation of joy.

In the beginning, there were times I felt so overwhelmed. I would even wake up in the middle of the night in a panic, all sweaty and hot with my heart racing a million miles a minute. It was so scary and almost as if I was watching my life from a distance, not actually a part of what was going on. I tried to ignore it at first, but things that had never bothered me started to weigh on my heart terribly. I was afraid to commit to anything and my emotions ran so high, making me feel like I could cry at the drop of a hat. What was happening to me? Was this a symptom of the brain tumor? Was it going to be better when the tumor was removed? Was I always going to feel so out of control and miserable?

I could see that panic was beginning to rule my mind: It was changing not only my life, but my personality as well. What was I going to do? How could I get through whatever I was going through? I was at a loss but soon realized that this was not just a battle of the mind: it was a battle for my heart and a fight for my life. I had to go into battle mode and fight for peace in my heart, clarity in my mind and victory over my circumstances. I began to question my responses to everything, look deep inside myself and think about all the promises that God had planted way down deep in my heart over the years.

As a Christian, I knew that the only thing I could do was go back to the basics. It seemed, as I was struggling, I had forgotten the most important aspect of dealing with anything... **What does the Lord say?** I really needed to set my thoughts on what He says about my circumstances. Once I got there, and reminded myself to go to the Lord, I decided I was not going to allow my life to be overtaken by fear. I made up my mind that I was going to reclaim His peace that passes all understanding and stand firm on God's word. I knew there was Joy in my heart and it didn't matter what I was going to go through. I was going to find that Joy and figure out how to restore its reign over my mind.

There is nothing like the Word of God to comfort and inspire us during difficult times. The world offers only empty solutions. Believe me: I have tried so many of them, but nothing compares to the promises and truths from God's Word. Many verses touch our hearts in different seasons of our lives, but I must say that my life verse has always stayed the same. It has reminded me time and time again, that even when I am weak, it is His Joy that gives me Strength.

Nehemiah 8:10 is not only a favorite verse, it has been a favorite song of mine since childhood. Perhaps, as you read it, you are singing it too.

"The Joy of the Lord is your Strength!" Nehemiah 8:10 (KJV)

Over the past few years I have discovered over and over just how important it is to have that foundation of Joy found in Nehemiah 8:10. When we don't, it is so easy to fall into that fear trap that causes us to become consumed with ourselves and our circumstances. Sometimes it is all we can think about. That is when things can really start to fall apart. I was in a place where I needed to reclaim my Joy. When bad things happen, we have to try to protect our heart. I knew that I was in a desperate place and needed the Strength that only comes from the Joy of the Lord.

Don't let me confuse you... I am not talking about happiness when I say that we need to be filled with the Joy of the Lord. Happiness and joy are very different things. Unhappiness can happen in any season of our lives. That does not mean in any way that something is wrong with us, or that the Joy of the Lord cannot be found in our heart. There have been times in my life that I have been very unhappy. I have lost close friends, missed important deadlines, struggled with chronic health issues, and, of course, undergone brain surgery. None of those things made me happy or gave me Joy, and I am sure that you can understand exactly what I am talking about. We all have our struggles that affect our happiness. When that happens, the most important thing we need to do is stand firm, and know that our Strength comes from the Joy of the Lord in our lives.

We must never let anything or anyone discourage us, or convince us, that we have lost our foundation of Joy. That is what the enemy wants us to believe. He wants us to be absolutely miserable. He wants to steal everything from us, including our Joy, but we need to stand on what the Lord tells us. God says how much He wants for us as His children, and that He will be the Strength in our lives, if we allow Him to be.

I am so thankful for the following verse in my life. I have it memorized and speak it out loud as a reminder of what I know the Lord wants for me, and what He wants for all of us. He wants us to have an abundant life.

I am come that they might have life, and that they might have it more abundantly. John 10:10b (KJV)

The truth is, the devil loves to see us unhappy and would love to steal our Joy in every negative situation, making us bitter, making us weak and making us believe that there is no hope. That is exactly what I was feeling as I battled against anxiety and panic. As I prepared for brain surgery, I needed to protect my heart, claiming John 10:10b whenever I became fearful of my future.

I needed the reminder that God wants us to have an abundant life, to build a firm foundation that can support me even through the tough stuff. When we are feeling down, that Joy that the Lord gives can overflow into our hearts and our minds when it is needed the most. That is exactly what I needed during so many different times throughout my recovery as I could feel my peace and my Joy slipping away.

Maybe you have been there, too? Have you ever felt as if everything in your life was falling apart? Maybe you are there now and it seems like you are stuck in the midst of a terrible situation or overwhelming trial. Perhaps you are thinking, there is no way that things could ever get better.

I am living proof that no matter what is going on in your life, God cares about it and He will help you through it. Isaiah 41:13 is a wonderful scripture to remind all of us of that we have help and God will take us by the hand to guide us through.

> *For I am the LORD your God who takes hold of your right hand and says to you, Do not fear; I will help you. Isaiah 41:13 (NIV)*

What a glorious promise and comfort to us as we struggle in our circumstances! Again, we have the promise that the Lord is there to help if we allow Him to. That was hard for me - allowing the Lord to help. Sometimes, I was what was standing in my own way. Part of my biggest issue was that I was afraid to let anyone know I was struggling. I needed encouragement and prayer, but I was afraid to ask for it. I can remember seeing post after post on my ministry prayer page of those who faithfully asked for prayer, but yet I remained silent about my own needs. Why was it so hard to admit I needed prayer? Maybe I didn't want to appear fearful or worried about my circumstances. Perhaps it was pride and I didn't want anyone to know I needed help because that would make me too vulnerable. It could be that I want to appear like I have everything under control. It is so hard to admit that we need help. That is true for so many of us.

When we are struggling, we look around and think we are surrounded by perfect people who need nothing; we feel they may judge our weakness. This is a monumental misconception! Because of our perception of other people's lives, we tend to try to put on a façade ourselves, making others think that everything is perfect in our lives as well. As I started to talk about what I was going through, it was very eye-opening to realize that there were NO perfect lives. We all live in the same sinful world, which means we are all going to have problems and trials of all kinds. We all need prayer for God's hand in our situation. Your trial may be different from mine, but the answers are all the same. We need to take it all to the Lord and ask Him for help, to surround ourselves with prayer warriors, to lift us up and encourage us. The truth is that we are all bruised and damaged by our circumstances. We just need to decide where we will go for our care.

I know that I have gone through times where I was embarrassed to share how I felt or what I was going through. Eventually though, I realized that I needed to put myself out there and that there should be NO need to question how it would look if I shared my fear or my lonely heart with others. As I look back, it really amazes me that when I noticed that someone else had a need, I was right there ready to intercede on their behalf, yet I was so worried how I would look if I asked for prayer in return. It was my pride that kept me from that blessing time and time again. The anxiety would rise within me and I would think to myself… What would they think of me? Would they consider me weak, weird or needy if I mentioned my plight? I was in a tough spot emotionally.

God really allowed me to be humbled, both by my needs and my circumstances. In spite of myself and my fears, I was able to experience the comfort and peace that passes all understanding as God brought one prayer warrior after another into my life - whether I asked or not (because He works in cool ways like that). They did not question my strength as a Christian or pity me for my circumstances; they simply lifted me up as a valued child of the King who needed a touch on her life. I learned through this experience that nothing strengthens our foundation of Joy like a team of prayer warriors flooding the throne on our behalf. Now when I have a need, the first people I go to for encouragement and prayer are my dear sisters and brothers in Christ. I have still stalled in neutral a few times due to my tendency to want to appear like I have everything under control, but with a gentle nudge the Lord reminds me how important it is to have an army that fights alongside you in the battle. We are never alone.

Even if you are not going through a cataclysmic event, just living life can sometimes be overwhelming. Perhaps the pressure you are under is causing a constant state of panic in your soul that it is stealing your Joy, and leaving you with little hope. Whatever it is that you are going through, God will bring you through it and give you peace. He will also send people alongside you, just as He did for me, to help you along the way.

When I was diagnosed with a brain tumor while I was already dealing with other health issues, I could feel my life spinning out of control. I didn't know what to deal with first, or how to face what I needed to do. All I could see was that once again, a major health crisis was going to steal my independence. The devil was trying to steal my Joy and take my peace by making me spin in circles.

It was a very hard time and sometimes quite scary. I had to give up so much. I knew it would be a very long time before I would be able to do many of the things I had been able to do in the past, assuming I was ever able to fully recover. I had no power over any part of the situation and felt totally helpless. That was when I started experiencing the fear and panic I shared earlier. That fear was making it even harder for me to know what was going on in my body, which actually made everything worse. I don't know if you are like this, but I am someone who likes to know how everything ends up and often read the end of a book first. In the same way, I wanted to know what was causing each of my symptoms. I was going through so many things, but had no idea what was causing any of it.

I had episodes of feeling faint, loss of vision and dizziness. My heart would beat out of control and make me feel sick. These symptoms were scary, and also extremely vague. I was so worried about what people would think of me if I went in to the doctor assuming something was really wrong, only to find out it was a panic attack. Even my jaw would ache and that made me question if I needed emergency treatment. Was it my heart? Was it symptoms caused by the brain tumor? Was it panic? It was a horrible position to be in, especially when I was trying to appear so strong. I really did not want to seem worried, or want to be worried for that matter. I would try to convince myself that I could get through this if I was tough enough.

Dealing with these chronic health issues has made me a "tough" girl, or at least that is how I liked to appear. It is definitely a learned state of mind. Over the years, I had developed a "never let 'em see you sweat" mentality. You may have heard that saying before as well. You don't let on that you are miserable, you don't show you are scared, and you certainly don't openly discuss any infirmities you may have. As I mentioned earlier, that mindset makes seeking encouragement or treatment very hard; you can't share the truth because you don't want anyone to know that you are struggling.

That mentality is now seemingly outdated. I have noticed that we are now living in a "you can share everything" society, but the ways of my youth still did not allow me to give out too many details of my private struggles. If someone would ask "How are you?", I simply responded "Doing OK, keeping busy, how are you?" After all, do they really want to know? Would I tell them that inside I am screaming or that I am miserable? Did they see any signs of panic as they looked into my eyes? Would it have even mattered?

I may have hidden it well from most people, but it was impossible to hide it from myself. I could see that panic and anxiety were starting to rule my life. I was in a desperate place but I just couldn't tell anybody. I was supposed to be an encourager. What would they think if I couldn't deal with things, or started asking others to encourage me? My fears of asking people for help and prayers were still an issue.

If you have been there, you know exactly what I am talking about. You just don't know what to do at that moment, and I know that my anxious heart was what was really keeping me from even thinking clearly. As we discussed earlier, I didn't want to appear weak or out of control. When you are in that kind of situation, how do you respond? Do you tell others you are struggling and risk appearing vulnerable, whiny or weak? Do you just keep it to yourself? I started to ask myself… "What would I tell someone else to do if I knew they were struggling?" I decided that I needed to take my own advice. I needed to ask for help and immediately go to the master physician. I had to understand what I was dealing with and take a look at what panic really was and what the good Lord had to say about dealing with it. I was desperate and needed help. The Lord already knew what I was going through and He would have all the answers I needed. But what was I dealing with? I knew I had a lot of health issues, but it became abundantly clear that I was struggling with anxiety as well. I was full of fear and starting to panic over even the most insignificant things. It had become quite debilitating and I needed answers. Why was I experiencing panic? What was panic anyway?

If you ask Google for a definition of panic, it will give you an explanation that goes something like this… Panic is described as a sudden overwhelming fear, with or without cause, that produces hysterical or irrational behavior that often spreads quickly through a group of people.

So, that explains a lot of what happens as you deal with anxiety and panic. Not only is panic overwhelming for the person experiencing it, panic is also contagious. When I read that, I began to think of some of the old sayings people use to repeat when I was a kid. Have you ever heard the one that says: "If Mama isn't happy, ain't nobody happy!" As a busy mom, I totally understand that saying. If Mom is in a panic, then everyone will be. The same thing goes in our churches, workplaces, communities, and in our country for that matter. When things don't go our way, it is easy to get overwhelmed and move into panic mode and even easier to bring everyone with us, creating an epidemic. As I started to panic about my situation, I could see how it was impacting my family. Imagine how panic can negatively affect our recovery during a major health crisis.

But, why was this happening? I discovered quite a few reasons. First, there are lot of things that can throw us into a panic. Too many things to do, misbehaving kids, preparing for a journey, an unfulfilling job, and on and on and on. While these things are stressful, we can rejoice in the fact that they are momentary. In those situations, we can confidently say "Tomorrow is another day", because those are examples of things that make us panic that we can do something about. We simply change our attitude or our response and those circumstances can change in a relatively short amount of time.

Another type of panic that happens is due to those things that we have no control over. These are the circumstances that can really send us reeling. Maybe it's a death of a loved one, an unexpected expense, or maybe, like me, it is something serious with your health. These things make us feel helpless, alone and fearful. It is because we know that we have no control over our situation.

For me, finding out I would need brain surgery was such a scary thing. Not because I hadn't experienced some terrible health scares.

In fact, the past 20 years had been full of physical challenges that I had no control over.

I longed to have children and God, in His goodness and mercy gave us 2 beautiful boys to raise. During both of my pregnancies, I experienced what they called spastic quadriplegia & was not able to care for my babies or myself when they were born. It was so hard to depend on others during a time when I, as a mom, was supposed to be the caregiver. I had this precious baby boy and was unable to be what he needed the most. I am so thankful for the Lord's hand on my life during those trying times. As I look back now, I can see how God was preparing me and showing me that He is the one in control and when we can't take care of ourselves or change our circumstances, HE gathers the troops and brings those who will fill in the gap during our time of need. That is why we need to ask for prayers and to let people know our needs.

As I was preparing for brain surgery, so many things were going through my head. How do I tell my children? What if I don't make it through the surgery? Will it affect my mind? Will I be able to do any of the things I could before the surgery? All of these questions and more were weighing heavily on my heart.

I knew it was going to be hard to get through the surgery and it would be a long, hard recovery. I definitely was in panic mode thinking about all the extreme possibilities. I asked myself… "How does one get ready for something like brain surgery?" I had a couple short weeks to prepare, and during that time, I tried to finish a lot of things that I had started… just in case. I could not believe how many "things" I had in my life that were still unfinished. That created even more anxiety as I kept feeling like I needed to take care of so much. I was feeling quite stressed and overwhelmed. Have you ever felt like that? Was I all alone?

As I was struggling to accomplish as much as I could, that was when the Lord stepped in and spoke to my heart. There would always be more things that needed to be accomplished, but the only thing that really mattered was my relationship with God, and time with family and friends. I realized that when we are going through trials, no matter what they are, we don't need to waste our time trying to catch up, we need to take that time to just be still. God was at work in my situation and gathered the prayer warriors and encouragers. They began to rally around us and our situation.

I was so amazed at the number of people who reached out to me and my family. It still brings a tear to my eye. I was so thankful that I let others in and sought the support of these great prayer warriors, even when it was hard to ask. What a blessing that was. What a comfort God gives us when we pray and when we have others praying for us. That is when God's peace that passes all understanding guards our hearts and minds. That peace helps us to focus and to release the anxiousness that wells up deep within, creating fear and stealing our peace.

Philippians 4:6-7 (NIV) reminds us:

> *Do not be anxious about anything, but in every situation, by prayer and petition, with thanksgiving, present your requests to God. And the peace of God, which transcends all understanding, will guard your hearts and your minds in Christ Jesus.*

One of the ways that God worked in my circumstances was to bring others in to help us out. So many people from all over were a light to our family during that time of preparation. I can never express how grateful I am for that. God is so GOOD! He has given me the blessing of a gracious and Godly family, including parents that are loving, kind and so generous with all they have, but, most importantly, with their time. They have been there every step of the way, encouraging me, inspiring me, escorting me and lifting me up before the King of Kings. All I had to do was mention a need and they would immediately stop everything they were doing and go to the Lord in prayer. I cannot tell you what a blessing that has been to me.

If you are going through a difficult time in your life, it is important to seek help and allow people to help you along the journey. Like we discussed earlier, it is hard to admit that you need help, but once you do, it blesses you and the one who comes alongside of you like nothing else can. Helping others, giving of yourself, and lifting people up in times of need is a high calling that makes a real difference in the lives of those around you. Asking for help was hard and receiving was something that I certainly needed to learn how to do. Letting others be blessed by allowing them to do for me and my family was an essential part of the healing process. It can be very difficult. A wonderful group of ladies from church came to my house to clean. I have to admit that I had a hard time and felt embarrassed as they scrubbed my toilet, mopped my floors and dusted my woodwork. What would they think about my messy bathroom or my filthy windows? My pride almost kept me from receiving a blessing and it also would have kept them from being a blessing. The truth is they didn't bat an eye at my dirty floors, dusty woodwork or my well used shower. They just went right to work. It hadn't been easy to allow these women to come in and clean my house, but the end result was a true, powerful blessing. Having a home that sparkled and smelled like springtime made me feel better; it brought me Joy and it was one less thing that I would have to think about.

Turning From Panic to Peace

God was definitely doing a big work in my life. As I was dealing with everything I was going through, there are times I felt so sad and I would even have moments that made me feel like I was losing the battle. That is when the Lord would intervene, reminding me again that He is there.

One of the hardest times for me was during one of my pre-surgical scans. I was sitting in my chilly (and ever so drab) hospital attire, for yet another MRI, when I felt an overwhelming panic come over me like never before. As the door slowly closed behind me, I waved goodbye to my husband in the waiting room and it hit me; I was all alone and NO ONE would be able to go with me. I became acutely aware of my surroundings. I saw the Emergency Exit and fleetingly thought to myself, how great it would be to just open the door and run as fast as I can away from the hospital. I could forget about the tumor, forget about the surgery and just run.

As that was going through my mind, I noticed one person after another came past and I slowly began to see my surroundings differently. I saw other hurting people that were most likely experiencing the same feelings of anxiety that I was. I stopped looking at the Exit and nervously started to smile and joke and ask how they were doing. Some opened up to share their story and others just smiled back. I was amazed at how the Lord had opened the opportunity for me to think about others when I had been so busy just thinking about myself. Even in my ugly and uncomfortable hospital gown, God found a way to touch my heart. As if that wasn't enough, I came home to message after message on my computer that encouraged me. God knew just what I needed to calm my anxious heart. I knew after that happened that to get through the surgery and recovery I needed to start looking at things in a different way. I had to stop focusing on my problems.

Focus on TRUTH

While praying about the upcoming surgery, I regrouped and began to change the way I was looking at my situation. I needed to stop concentrating on the problems and letting my thoughts take me to worrisome and dark places about my situation. I needed to stop thinking about the "What ifs" and begin to focus on what I knew to be truth. We can all do this because the truth does not change from problem to problem or person to person. What is the truth?

Here are three simple things I KNEW as TRUTH:

1. This was happening.
2. It was going to be hard.
3. God was in control.

When we go through situations that are beyond our control, we get so consumed with our circumstances that we forget to acknowledge those simple truths and fail to realize that we are not in control. What is the absolute truth about our lives?

1. The TRUTH is that our days are already numbered.

Psalm 139:16 (NIV) reminds us of that truth...

> *Your eyes saw my unformed body; all the days ordained for me were written in your book, before one of them came to be.*

It might seem a little morbid, but it was comforting to know that how long I will live had already been decided before I was even born. That simple truth took the pressure off: Nothing could be gained by panicking over whether I would survive the brain tumor and the brain surgery to rid me of them, because it had already been written in God's book of life. I had NO CHOICE but to give it all over to the Lord and trust in His plan for my life. It was not easy, but I really needed to trust in His promises and believe that regardless of what has already been decided about my life here, I have an eternal hope and a future with Christ in heaven. Again, I turned to the verse I was always sharing with my kids at church. Jeremiah 29:11 was a simple reminder of what the Lord has planned for me...

> *For I know the plans I have for you," declares the LORD, "plans to prosper you and not to*

harm you, plans to give you hope and a future.
Jeremiah 29:11 (**NIV**)

As you are reading this book today, may it remind you as well that no matter what is going on in your life, your story has already been written. We need to try to let go of our fear and follow the path that God has laid before us. Sometimes that path leads us over a rocky road, but we can remember these two things:

1. We are not alone.
2. We need not fear.

A verse that reminds me of this and has comforted and blessed my heart so much during tough times has been Deuteronomy 31:8. Sometimes, we just need a little reminder...

The LORD himself goes before you and will be with you; he will never leave you nor forsake you. Do not be afraid; do not be discouraged.
Deuteronomy 31:8 (**NIV**)

If you are going through something today and it feels as if there is no one beside you, let me assure you that you are wrong. God is ALWAYS there!

I have been so thankful for God's promise in that verse to never leave me. I can recall many times that I felt all alone, and even the fear I experienced as I was going through the many MRI scans that I needed. Not being a fan of tight places, I relied on God to help me through each and every scan. I can remember crying out to the Lord to just get me past the test. Some of you may be thinking, "buck up girlfriend, an MRI is no big deal", especially when you consider all of the other things I had to go through, but for me, it was very hard. When you are slightly claustrophobic, it feels like you are suffocating and like you will never make it through. It is also very hard to stay still for such a long time when you have a body that likes to move and tremor all of the time. Talk about PANIC!

I would pray every time that I had to have a scan that God would give me peace like never before. If you have ever had an MRI, you probably know exactly what I am talking about. For those of you who have not… Picture this: You are on a very uncomfortable table and slowly inserted into a very narrow tube that seems to be barely big enough to fit a small child. The air circulates around you and blows in your face, stealing your breath away as you try to remain calm. I knew that the scan was only temporary but something inside of me just needed the comfort that only the Lord can give.

It was during these times that I would sing out God's promises. I, of course, would sing them in my head because you are not allowed to move in the MRI. When I would get stressed and start singing out loud, they would have to repeat the scan. That was something I really tried to avoid with everything in me. I loved singing scripture songs that I had hidden in my heart and was always encouraged by the song Chris Tomlin sings that says "I know who goes before me, I know who stands behind, the God of Angel armies is always by my side." I just love that little reminder. I would sing it over and over in the MRI to get me through. It really worked to focus on the Lord's presence and calmed me from the inside out. I knew that not only is God right there with me, just as the scripture says, but He has gone before me and He will come behind me, prodding me to victory!

I must say that through all of the MRI's, lab tests, and even the surgery, there is one thing that I know for sure: if I did not have the Joy of the Lord in my life, I would not have been able to receive the peace that He gave me. I would soon learn that it was only through that foundation of joy in my heart that I would be able to get through the rest of my treatment and recovery. That does not mean that it was smooth sailing and everything went well; frankly, it was a very rocky road to recovery. I often experienced physical trials and situations that brought about anxiety and panic like I can't even express, but every day my heart was calmed by leaning on the Lord's promises.

You may not be going through brain surgery, but, perhaps there is a situation in your life that is stealing your Joy. You need to turn to the Lord like never before to keep this from happening.

It really is like this saying I have heard so many times before:

If you have NO JOY, you will have NO PEACE, but if you KNOW JOY, you can KNOW PEACE.

Without peace, we tend to panic. Once I knew what was hindering my preparation for surgery and recovery, I knew I needed to tackle it step-by-step. That brings us to each of the lessons I learned when preparing for BRAIN SURGERY, and the message I would like to share… DON'T PANIC!

DON'T <u>P</u>LANT SEEDS OF DOUBT

When we are going through a tough time in our lives, our biggest problem often has nothing to do with WHAT we are going through, but everything to do with HOW we react to what we are going through. Sometimes, we can be our own worst enemy and actually allow ourselves to be taken down even further by what we are thinking and what we are saying about our circumstances. That brings us to the first thing I learned during my surgery and recovery.

<u>DON'T PLANT SEEDS OF DOUBT!</u>

We have all heard the saying "Sticks and stones can break your bones, but words can never hurt you". With no offense to the person who started saying that, I would have to disagree wholeheartedly. We are reminded time and time again by God that words are very powerful and those words can be so damaging, both to ourselves and others.

The tongue has the power of life and death...
Proverbs 18:21a **(NIV)**

Do not let any unwholesome talk come out of your mouths, but only what is helpful for building others up according to their needs, that it may benefit those who listen. Ephesians 4:29 **(NIV)**

My very wise mother has told me time and time again that I can choose to speak LIFE or speak DEATH over any situation and that it was totally up to me. She would never belittle my circumstances or tell me to pretend everything was OK. She was telling me that I was the one who could choose to proclaim victory or proclaim defeat over my circumstances, and whatever my choice was, that is what I should expect to experience in that situation.

You see, a lot of what we think about ourselves, or our circumstances, is important. If I am experiencing difficulties trying to win an award and keep telling myself, "I am never going to get it", "I am just not smart enough", or "I never win anything, so how can I get this?", then pretty soon, that is exactly what I believe about what I am going through. Eventually I start to think, "Why bother?" It is never going to work out the way I need it to, so I give up. I needed to stop planting seeds of doubt in my life and start speaking truth and victory.

I know that when I put it that way, it makes it sound so easy. Believe me… I know from experience, it is NOT! I know how hard it is to be positive when everything around you is negative. When you are hearing a scary diagnosis, going through a painful divorce, experiencing family or financial troubles, or, maybe, the loss of a loved one, all you feel at that moment is defeat and despair. It is very hard to look on the bright side, and even harder to speak good about a devastating situation. At this point, the seeds of doubt are not only planted, but they are starting to take over your life's garden.

After my surgery, I tried so hard to keep a bright, cheery and positive outlook on everything that was going on. My body did not respond well to the surgery. I had lost all motor function and experienced spastic tremors that stole my ability to even hold a hand for comfort. I was starting at square one and, like a small child, I would have to redevelop my skills, one step at a time. I had to relearn everything, and I celebrated every milestone. You would not believe the joy that overcomes you, the first time you are allowed to sit on the toilet without someone holding you up straight so you don't fall off. (I know TMI… but I wanted to share some of my biggest everyday victories).

It has certainly been a very long recovery. Every day I stood on the victory that I know I can have in Christ Jesus. I knew that on my own I could do nothing, but with God, all things are possible. I had to believe that these "shaky" hands were going to, once again, do the Lord's work steadily. I was going to proclaim that over my entire body every single day.

As hard as I tried to always look on the bright side, there was a certain day that the devil got tired of my cheery disposition and decided to throw me a curveball that I did not see coming. I was undergoing intensive physical, occupational and memory therapy. Learning to walk, move, remember… All of the things we take for granted every day. It was hard and exhausting, both physically and mentally, yet I was going to continue to keep my eyes on Jesus and smile, even when I didn't feel like it, and laugh when I really felt like crying.

Just as I was being wheeled out of my therapy session, feeling hot, sweaty and like a wet noodle, I saw a familiar face standing near the front desk. Even though I was exhausted, I mustered up a smile and sat up straight in my wheelchair to say hello. As I did, I saw the scowl on her face and heard the words come straight out of her mouth that hit my heart like an arrow… "So, you're still in a wheelchair?" I know those words may not sound bad to you, but to me they were just enough to water those seeds of doubt in my mind and start them growing.

I did not have a response, but I do remember my encouraging

therapist leaning down and whispering in my ear "She has no idea" as she gently touched my shoulder. Her words were a comfort, but I could feel the tears welling up inside as my husband pushed me onto the elevator. As soon as the doors closed, tears just started to pour. My husband had no idea what had just happened and could only listen to me as every doubt about my life, my recovery and my motivation came pouring out of my mouth. I started to wonder what was wrong with me. Why was I still in the wheelchair? It had been 6 months since my brain surgery. I knew several people who had gone through brain surgery and they were doing great. Had I not been trying hard enough? Was I being lazy? Was I not doing everything I could to move forward and be a viable part of my life, my family and my community? I felt stuck between where I was and what I began to think about myself.

Thankfully, I have a very encouraging husband and family. They had been with me during the entire recovery, and gently reminded me of how far I had come. I was also reminded that I was not going to go very far if I talked about my situation that way. My mother's words started to echo in my head. "You can speak life, or speak death over your situation."

What happened that made me forget that? As I started to replay the day in my head, I started to rethink the words that were said to me. The truth is, I am sure my friend never meant them to be negative. I was in a vulnerable place, and the devil saw an opportunity to knock me down. It was my mindset that needed to change, and I was the one who had to get rid of my STINKIN' THINKIN'!

As we speak about our circumstances or about ourselves, we need to remember that our lives will go exactly where our words say they will. You have to think positively and you have to speak positively. The best way I know to speak life is by claiming God's Word. When we do that, it will encourage and lift us up no matter what we are going through. That is the only thing that will give us power over our circumstances. When we do that, we are claiming VICTORY over our lives! We need to look for good and start proclaiming that good news in our situation and like my mother says… Speak life, don't speak death!

Jesus came to give us an abundant life full of hope for a better tomorrow. Don't let the devil steal your JOY by planting doubt in your heart and mind!

Remember what the Word of God says the devil's goal is:

> *The thief comes only to steal and kill and destroy. I came that they may have life and have it abundantly. John 10:10* **(NIV)**

When I am going through a situation where I feel that I am starting to panic or plant seeds of doubt, I look for encouragement from God's Word. I try to look at those in the Bible who have gone through difficult or confusing times, and try to study how they got through them.

- Did they turn to the Lord and plead with Him for help?
- Did they act strong and try to get through it themselves?
- Did God send someone their way to help them along?
- Were they obedient?
- What was the outcome?

As I look into the scriptures I see the story of Mary, Mother of Jesus…

Luke 1:26-33 (NIV)

> *In the sixth month of Elizabeth's pregnancy, God sent the angel Gabriel to Nazareth, a town in Galilee, to a virgin pledged to be married to a man named Joseph, a descendant of David. The virgin's name was Mary. The angel went to her and said, "Greetings, you who are highly favored! The Lord is with you."*

> *Mary was greatly troubled at his words and wondered what kind of greeting this might be. But the angel said to her, "Do not be afraid, Mary; you have found favor with God. You will conceive and give birth to a son, and you are to call him Jesus. He will be great and will be called the Son of the Most High. The Lord God will give him the throne of his father David, and he will reign over Jacob's descendants forever; his kingdom will never end."*

Imagine this young girl, probably around 14-years-old, just a baby herself, being approached by an angel (that in itself could cause a bit of a panic if you ask me). The angel proceeds to tell her that she was chosen to be the mother of God's son.

I need to stop right there for a minute to take this in…

- She is only 14.
- She is NOT married.
- Did the Lord understand the times; the people; the culture?
- Did He know that she could be stoned?

Of course He did! There are so many questions that go through my mind, and I wonder if any doubts came to Mary as she was told these things. We know that she was faithful by her response.

Luke 1:38 (NIV)

> *"I am the Lord's servant," Mary answered. "May your word to me be fulfilled." Then the angel left her.*

Throughout the story of her pregnancy, we see that she was never overtaken by panic or seeds of doubt, even in the worst of circumstances. She is quite an example of a trusting woman.

Every year in the Christmas story we hear about the LONG journey to Bethlehem on the back of a donkey. I must confess, I have never ridden a donkey, but have been on a horse and cannot even fathom how she made it. Remember, Mary is PREGNANT, in fact, it says she was great with child in Luke 2:4-5 (KJV). The story continues...

Luke 2:4-5 (KJV)

> *So Joseph also went up from Nazareth in Galilee to Judea, to the City of David called Bethlehem, since he was from the house and line of David. To be taxed with Mary his espoused wife, being great with child.*

They have to make the long trip to Bethlehem which is about 65 miles. I don't know about you, but my family rarely makes it 65 miles in a car before some kind of complaining starts. Mary and Joseph's trip would have taken days. However, even during such a long, hard trip, we still never hear anything about how she was scared or nervous. WOW! In fact, as we read, there seems to be a peace that passes all understanding over the entire story. If it was me, I would have questioned so many things...

- Was she going to make the trip?
- Was she going to have to stop to deliver along the way?

We do know they made it to Bethlehem, and that when they got there Mary was in labor and ready to deliver. Because of the census, Bethlehem was full of people. They had nowhere to stay, and the baby was coming. This situation must have been very distressing. It definitely would have put me into panic mode. These days, we get upset if the hotel room smells funny or the bed isn't made right.

They did not even have a room, but we see where they ended up.

Luke 2:7 (KJV)

And she brought forth her firstborn son, and wrapped him in swaddling clothes, and laid him in a manger; because there was no room for them in the inn.

What a journey she had and what a blessing it was for her to deliver a beautiful baby boy just as the angel proclaimed. She became the mother of Jesus and because of God's plan, we can be saved. God is so good and so faithful. He has promised us that no matter what is happening in our lives, He is with us. If you are going through a difficult time, and it seems like a long hard road, think about Mary's journey and be inspired by all that the Lord does to fulfill His plan for our lives. Mary's journey also encourages me to trust fully in the Lord's plan for my life, especially when I am in the midst of the storm.

Prayer for a doubting heart…

Dear Heavenly Father, thank you for being the Father of TRUTH! Today I choose to completely trust in you. I give you all of my doubts about myself and my circumstances. I will stand on the foundation of joy that you have built for me. I will believe the things that you say about me.

I am your child!

You are always with me!

You have a plan for my life!

Thank you for your love and your peace that passes all understanding.

I realized that with each lesson I learned, I needed to have a spiritual check-up so that I could know exactly what I was dealing with and attack each symptom I had with effective treatments and just the right prescription. You can also answer the following questions and look up the scriptures to see what the Lord tells us to do for each diagnosis.

DIAGNOSIS: PLANTING SEEDS OF DOUBT

SYMPTOMS: Insecurity, Confusion, Disbelief, Distrust, Skepticism, Paranoia, Fearful, Unsettled, General Malaise (Icky feeling)

TREATMENT: To overcome self-doubt, concentrate on the things that you know and focus on speaking life over your situation. It is also imperative to surround yourself with people who are positive and supportive, people who keep reminding us of who God says we are and what He says about our situation.

PRESCRIPTION: (This needs to be done DAILY) Speak life over your situation and remember who you are as a child of God.

SIDE EFFECTS: May increase your ability to look on the bright side of every situation. USE WITH CARE as you develop your Christ-like attitude and apply it to your life.

<u>CHECKUP</u>

1. What kind of struggles are you facing today?

2. Are you Planting Seeds of Doubt over your situation?

3. What do you think you need to do to get rid of your Stinkin' Thinkin'?

4. What does the Bible tell you about your life in John 10:10?

5. What steps will you take to start speaking LIFE over your situation?

WORDS OF ENCOURAGEMENT: NO MORE DOUBTS!

WHEN YOU ARE DOUBTING EVERYTHING... FOCUS ON TRUTH!

The LORD is my rock, my fortress and my deliverer; my God is my rock, in whom I take refuge, my shield and the horn of my salvation, my stronghold. Psalm 18:2 (NIV)

As for God, his way is perfect: The LORD's word is flawless; he shields all who take refuge in him. Psalm 18:30 (NIV)

You will keep in perfect peace those whose minds are steadfast, because they trust in you. Isaiah 26:3 (NIV)

WHEN YOU ARE DOUBTING YOURSELF...
BE CONFIDENT IN CHRIST!

Though an army besiege me, my heart will not fear; though war break out against me, even then I will be confident. Psalm 27:3 (NIV)

For God has not given us a spirit of fear and timidity, but of power, love, and self-discipline. 2 Timothy 1:7 (NLT)

Finally, be strong in the Lord and in his mighty power. Ephesians 6:10 (NIV)

WHEN YOU ARE DOUBTING GOD...
SEE HIS FAITHFULNESS!

But the Lord is faithful, and he will strengthen you and protect you from the evil one. 2 Thessalonians 3:3 (NIV)

The LORD thy God in the midst of thee is mighty; he will save, he will rejoice over thee with joy; he will rest in his love, he will joy over thee with singing. Zephaniah 3:17 (KJV)

Look at the birds of the air; they do not sow or reap or store away in barns, and yet your heavenly Father feeds them. Are you not much more valuable than they? Matthew 6:26 (NIV)

Cast all your anxiety on Him, because He cares for you. 1 Peter 5:7 (NIV)

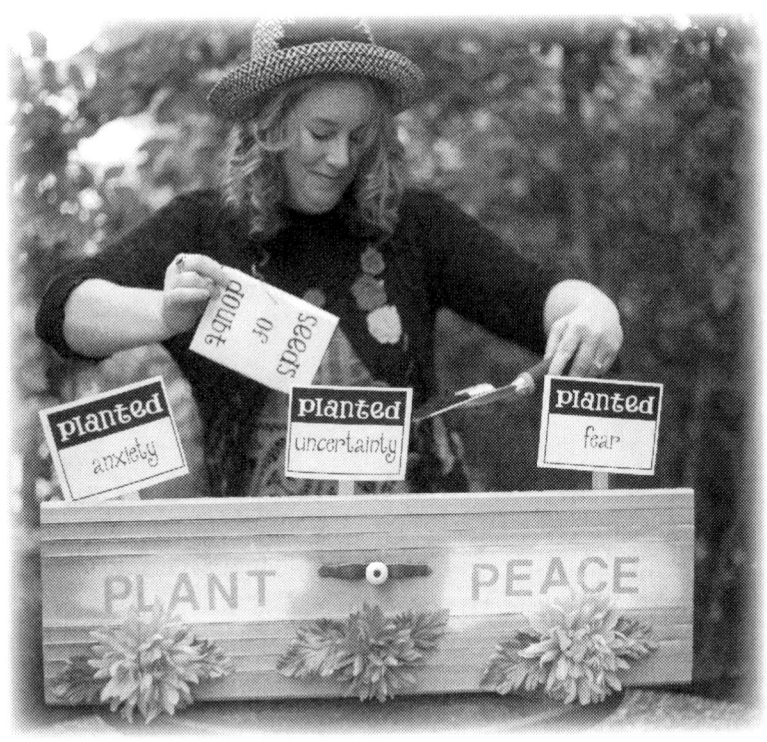

Be careful what you are planting in your garden of life!

DON'T BE ANXIOUS

Another very important lesson I learned throughout my recovery was Don't Be Anxious! Anxiety is a very real emotion. When we are anxious, our heart beats faster, our breathing is very shallow, and we may even start to feel sick to our stomach. I am not talking about butterflies before a performance or nervousness about an exam. I am talking about the overwhelming anxiety, or should I say FEAR, that takes our entire body captive and keeps us from experiencing the blessings that God has in store for us even during the darkest times.

Have you ever experienced anxiety or a panic attack? Perhaps you have had circumstances in which you have been overwhelmed with anxiousness or fear, and that fear caused you to act or react inappropriately to the situation you were in. When we are afraid, we tend to lose our ability to make good choices in regard to our surroundings. I have experienced anxiety at times that was actually crippling and literally made me feel as if I was having a heart attack. It is very real.

As we take a look at ourselves and how we react to trying situations, we start to realize that anxiety is consuming and that the only way we can deal with it is by giving it to the Lord and arming ourselves against those thoughts and ideas that not only instill fear and anxiety, but create an environment of defeat.

I can remember experiencing fear at a young age in varying degrees, but the majority of my anxiety has been associated with my health. I told you about my "never let 'em see you sweat" mentality earlier in this book, and that thought process has created some problems in my mind and how I deal with fear and anxiety. That keep it to yourself mindset offers even more issues as problems arise. After all, I certainly wouldn't want anyone to know that I was feeling anxious, or that I was full of fear about anything. So, in my mind, it wasn't just the fear of what was happening, I was also afraid that someone might find out that I was fearful and anxious about the situation. It sounds kind of silly now, but that in itself created more anxiety. It was definitely a snowball effect.

The truth is, that I went through a time when I was afraid of almost everything. I was only comfortable going places when surrounded by those who were my safety net (my parents, husband and a couple of friends). I was a very social person and longed to just get out and see people, but I had let the enemy get inside my head and convince me that things were not what they really were. I felt as if I was a prisoner in my own mind and my thoughts usually wondered something like this...

- What if I have a fainting spell in public?
- What if I fall when I go to the store?
- What if I can't remember the things I need to say?
- What if I cannot do things the way that I did before?
- What if I lose my vision while I am out?

My thoughts continued to overwhelm me with these questions and many more until I began to speak against them. After all, the Bible tells us NOT to be ANXIOUS about anything.

Philippians 4:6-7 (**NIV**)

> **Do not be anxious about anything, but in every situation, by prayer and petition, with thanksgiving, present your requests to God. And the peace of God which transcends all understanding shall Guard your hearts and your minds in Christ Jesus.**

Once again, the Lord reminded me to look to him, and I knew that in order to combat my anxious heart, I would need to focus on His truth. The truth is that even if any of those things that I was so worried about actually happened to me, it did not change the fact that GOD IS IN CONTROL! It was hard, but I got through that time with the Lord's help. Just like the verse says, He gave me His peace that would guard my heart and my mind from all of the negative things swirling in them.

Another verse that was comforting showed me that even though I am surrounded by difficult and scary things, there is NOTHING that can separate me from Christ. It offers comfort and truth. If you are going through a time of anxiousness about yourself, or your situation… REMEMBER THIS VERSE!

Romans 8:35-39 (NIV)

> **Who shall separate us from the love of Christ? Shall trouble or hardship or persecution or famine or nakedness or danger or sword? As it is written: "For your sake we face death all day long; we are considered as sheep to be**

slaughtered." No, in all these things we are more than conquerors through him who loved us. For I am convinced that neither death nor life, neither angels nor demons, neither the present nor the future, nor any powers, neither height nor depth, nor anything else in all creation, will be able to separate us from the love of God that is in Christ Jesus our Lord.

Now as I look back over my recovery, I laugh because I cannot believe some of the things that made me anxious. One of the funniest times I can recall is from a very busy day, as I was recovering in the hospital rehab program. Picture this…

I am sitting in my wheelchair, slumped over in exhaustion, almost ready for bed. It had been a very long day. I had begun a rigorous routine in the hospital during a very important part of my recovery. After being in therapy sessions on and off since 7:30 in the morning, I had finally settled into my room, waiting somewhat impatiently for my supper to be delivered. Medication, combined with the intensive and long therapy sessions made me so hungry that, if I could have, I would have eaten my own shoe.

If you have had any experiences in the hospital, you know that schedules are extremely important. When things do not happen at the time they are supposed to, it can really throw you off and make you even more anxious than you were before. I was a nervous wreck and so hungry. It was time for dinner. After what seemed like a lifetime of waiting, someone finally delivered my meal. I can honestly say, at that moment in time, it was the best thing I had ever smelled. ONE BIG PROBLEM… they just dropped it off and left it on the tray in front of me, saying that someone would be right in to help me. I became so anxious about the entire situation, I thought I would explode.

Since I was unable to feed myself at that time, I had to try to be patient and wait. I was at that point in my recovery when I needed to rely on others. I waited and waited... No one came. The wonderful smell of this classic comfort food (Spaghetti -my favorite) was wafting in front of me. With an overwhelming angst, I decided that I was just going to help myself. I went for it, knocked off the lid and dove right in. No special utensils, no one to help me hold the fork or help me hit my mouth. Within minutes, I was covered head-to-toe with spaghetti. It was also all over the bed, wheelchair, and floor. I must have looked totally ridiculous as I tried and tried to get something in my mouth. The small amounts I was able to eat did not quench my hunger at all.

It was at that moment I looked up and saw the nurse peeking into the room with an expression that can only be described as hilarious. She saw me covered in spaghetti sauce and noodles. It was priceless I am sure, but she never flinched. She just simply looked at me, smiled and said "Okay then, I'll be right back with another tray." I am sure she burst into laughter the moment she hit the nurses' station. I felt kind of like a kid who got caught doing something wrong and was sitting in the principal's office.

I was so hungry and I became so anxious because one of my most basic needs was not being met. Had I forgotten to give it to the Lord? It sure made me think... Do I do that in other situations? Did I allow my anxious heart (and hungry tummy) to push me into an unsafe situation? Perhaps in my anxiousness, I became irrational in my thought process, forgetting that God is in control. I dove in, haphazardly trying to do things in my own power and made a mess. I know it is only spaghetti but it sure made me think about my over-reactions to other things in my life.

All throughout the Bible, we read God's message to not be anxious about anything because He has got it covered.

Looking in the Word, I think about Gideon and the situation he was faced with in Judges 7. He had a pretty good sized army of about 32,000 men when the Lord told him there were too many. The Lord said to Gideon in verse 3 to send home all of the men who were afraid. Surprisingly, only 10,000 men stayed. Can you imagine how that must have made Gideon feel about his army? He lost 22,000 men and he hadn't even gone to war yet. He was going to have to defeat the large camp of the Midianites with only 10,000 soldiers.

As if that wasn't distressing enough, the Lord then told Gideon he still had too many men. He told him that He would thin them out even more and asked Gideon to take them to the water. Can you imagine the anxiety Gideon must have felt knowing that he was losing even more men? Isn't it easier to win a battle with a larger, stronger army?

At the waterfront, the Lord separated the men once again by instructing Gideon to only keep those men who cupped the water in their hands and lapped it like a dog. That only included 300 men! So now the army that would attack the Midianites went from 32,000 down to 300. That is quite a difference, and frankly, pretty scary for Gideon.

Of course, Gideon was anxious and had to look to the Lord to find out what to do. How do I know that Gideon was feeling some anxiety about the situation? Take a look at verses 8-11 when the Lord tells him what to do.

Judges 7:9-11(NIV)

> ***During that night the Lord said to Gideon, "Get up, go down against the camp, because I am going to give it into your hands. If you are afraid to attack, go down to the* camp with your servant Purah and listen to what they are saying. Afterward, you will be encouraged to attack the camp."**

So, Gideon listens to the Lord and snuck down to the camp to listen to what they were saying.

Judges 7:13-15 (NIV)

Gideon arrived just as a man was telling a friend his dream. "I had a dream," he was saying. "A round loaf of barley bread came tumbling into the Midianite camp. It struck the tent with such force that the tent overturned and collapsed."

His friend responded, "This can be nothing other than the sword of Gideon son of Joash, the Israelite. God has given the Midianites and the whole camp into his hands." When Gideon heard the dream and its interpretation, he bowed down and worshiped.

Now, Gideon knew that the Lord had the entire situation in His hands and that calmed his anxious heart. They went on to defeat the large camp of Midianites with only 300 soldiers by being obedient and keeping their eyes on the Lord.

We don't have to allow anxiety to rule our lives or our circumstances. We need to fix our eyes on the Lord, just like Gideon, to win whatever battle we are going through.

Looking unto Jesus the author and finisher of our faith; who for the joy that was set before him endured the cross, despising the shame, and is set down at the right hand of the throne of God.
Hebrews 12:2 (KJV)

As I recall my story from the hospital, it certainly wasn't anything earth shattering or Gideon-like. In fact, I usually get a big chuckle when I think about it, but truly, as I look back to those feelings of anxiousness and hunger, I realize that it made me learn another valuable lesson in relation to the anxiety I was experiencing. If I hunger for the things of Christ, I will be blessed. My worldly anxiousness will be calmed and I will want even more of the things of God which bring peace. That does not include an anxious heart. How do I know this? I read it in God's Word.

> **Blessed are those who hunger and thirst for righteousness.** *Matthew 5:6* **(NIV)**

Prayer for an anxious heart...

> *Dear Heavenly Father, thank you for the gift of PEACE! Today I choose to give you every part of this ANXIOUS Heart. I look to the truth about my situation and lay all of my worries at your feet. I will remember how you have made me.*
>
> *I am made whole!*
>
> *I am made NEW!*
>
> *You have made a way for me!*
>
> *Thank you, Heavenly Father for your gift of peace that comforts me each and every day.*

DIAGNOSIS: ANXIETY/FEAR

SYMPTOMS: Fear, Panic, Nervousness, Problems Sleeping, Shortness of Breath, General Malaise (Icky feeling)

TREATMENT: To overcome ANXIETY, focus on the TRUTH and surround yourself with people who help you remember who you are in Christ and what He says about your situation. When you start to feel symptoms of anxiety or fear, claim the verses in the Words of Encouragement on the next page.

PRESCRIPTION: Put on your SONGLASSES: Fix your eyes on Jesus and change your focus to God, claiming for yourself His peace that passes all understanding in your life. (I tell you the truth...It's hard, but the more you do it, the more you will experience His peace)

SIDE EFFECTS: You will experience the feeling of calm in every aspect of your life. Your heart will also be blessed by God's peace that passes all understanding.

<u>CHECKUP</u>

1. Are you feeling ANXIOUS or FEARFUL about your life today?

2. How are those fears affecting your situation?

3. What do you think you can do to calm your ANXIOUS heart?

4. What does the Bible tell you about your situation in Philippians 4:6-7?

5. What is the truth about your situation that we see in Romans 8:35-39?

WORDS OF ENCOURAGEMENT: FOR PERFECT PEACE!

WHEN YOU ARE FEELING ANXIOUS ABOUT ANYTHING… TRUST IN THE LORD!

Trust in the LORD with all your heart and lean not on your own understanding. Proverbs 3:5 (NIV)

Cast your cares on the LORD and he will sustain you; he will never let the righteous be shaken. Psalm 55:22 (NIV)

Even though I walk through the darkest valley, I will fear no evil, for you are with me; your rod and your staff, they comfort me. Psalm 23:4 (NIV)

WHEN YOU ARE FEELING FEARFUL... BE CONFIDENT IN THE LORD!

So do not fear, for I am with you; do not be dismayed, for I am your God. I will strengthen you and help you; I will uphold you with my righteous right hand. Isaiah 41:10 (NIV)

Peace is what I leave with you; it is my own peace that I give you. I do not give it as the world does. Do not be worried and upset; do not be afraid. John 14:27 (NIV)

Say to those with fearful hearts, "Be strong, do not fear; your God will come, he will come with vengeance; with divine retribution he will come to save you. Isaiah 35:4 (NIV)

For the Spirit God gave us does not make us timid, but gives us power, love and self-discipline. 2 Timothy 1:7 (NIV)

WHEN YOU START TO WORRY... GIVE IT ALL TO THE LORD!

"Do not let your hearts be troubled. You believe in God; believe also in me." John 14:1 (NIV)

LESSON THREE

DON'T BE <u>N</u>EGATIVE

One of the most important, and possibly the most difficult, lessons I learned throughout my recovery was the necessity of a GOOD and POSITIVE OUTLOOK, no matter what you are facing. If you allow yourself to get into a negative mode, it is so difficult to restore a positive thought process. Remember from our first lesson that our lives will go in the direction of our words and, if our words are negative, our whole attitude and outlook will be negative as well.

I will let you in on a little secret… The devil would like nothing more than to steal your joy and give you a negative attitude about your situation. He knows that we cannot heal if our heart is broken and our eyes are fixed on how miserable we are. He wants us to be overwhelmed by our circumstances and overcome by bad emotions that leave us tired, motionless and unmotivated.

I am sure we all know someone who has been broken by the winds of life and has become a rather Gloomy Gus (That's a technical term). A GLOOMY GUS is someone who sees bad in everything because the negative attitude has grown so greatly that they are consumed with pointing out what is wrong with everything. Even though the sun may be shining, they complain about a storm that might come or even one that may have been there a while back. When our minds are set in negative mode, we can never find joy in anything. When you are going through a hard time, the last thing you should do is be around someone who is negative, because it is so contagious.

A Gloomy Gus is able to make even the best situations seem like mucking out the stalls. My husband likes to call that being a "FUN SPONGE". (Someone who can take the fun out of anything.) Not only is there no fun for them, they make it so there is no fun, no peace, and no happiness for anyone else either. It is not only a sad life, but I am sure it is a rather lonely one too.

When we are going through a tough time physically, emotionally or spiritually, we can tend to be drawn to music, movies and even people (fun sponges) who will feed our negative emotions and actually send us deeper and deeper into a darkness spurred on by a negative attitude.

It is not my intention to tell you that you should never feel sad or discouraged in your battle, or that listening to a good ol' sad song is bad for you. (Because I know that "Sad songs say so much!" LOL) Our feelings are real and justified, but it is our attitude that will either help us or hinder us as we make our way through our circumstances.

Day by day, throughout my recovery, I would try with all of my heart to have a good attitude. It can be very difficult when you are experiencing hard times, but I knew that if I did not focus on the positives and fix my eyes on the things of God, that I would be simply miserable.

You might be saying to yourself (or to me at this moment) that a good attitude is easier said than done. At certain times I would agree and even say... You got that right! I have experienced so many times when I really had to check my attitude and change my point of view.

One of those times, and one of the hardest things that I had to deal with, was watching the world around me go on like it always had, and I could only be a spectator. I was in a place where I felt stuck and I was totally dependent on others. Do you ever feel like that? You are a spectator in your own life? Months into my recovery, I started looking through Facebook, viewing all of my friends' pages and admiring beautiful images of their cheery lives. I saw post after post of vacations, dinners out with family and friends, canning, crafting and doing laundry (yes, I even romanticized doing the laundry). They were going to shows with their families and participating in school activities. At first I was thrilled to be included in their life celebrations, but the more I saw of these wonderful posts, the more I was drawn into a deep funk full of jealousy and even bitterness. I remember some of the posts that upset me were not even big things. It could be a simple post about how much they had accomplished by 7am when I was still waiting for someone to help me brush my teeth.

There you have it… I had entered the poor Pitiful Pearl phase of my recovery. I kept feeling sorry for myself and for the fact that I wasn't able to do any of those things with my family. I started to think that my boys and my husband were being cheated by having a mother and wife who was unable to participate in life, to take them places and do the kind of things that other families did regularly. The devil, who is the father of lies, was able to convince me that I was not who the Lord says I am. I was measuring my worth through what I was physically able to do and that was causing me to believe that I was worthless. I had to once again get rid of that "stinkin' thinkin'" and remember the TRUTH about what my Lord says about me.

He says…

> *I am chosen of God, holy and dearly loved.*
> *Colossians 3:12* **(NIV)**

It did not take long at all for the Lord to open my eyes to my situation and for me to check my attitude and change it. I needed to take a look at what I was putting in front of me and even allowing inside my mind, in order to start renewing my mind and changing my attitude. It was at that time he gave me one of the verses I now measure everything against. Philippians 4:8 is what I am claiming as the theme verse to this book because if you truly follow what it says… You will live in peace and I guarantee you will have a good and positive attitude and outlook, even during the darkest of times.

> *Finally, brethren, whatsoever things are true, whatsoever things are honest, whatsoever things are just, whatsoever things are pure, whatsoever things are lovely, whatsoever things are of good report; if there be any virtue, and if there be any praise, think on these things. Philippians 4:8* **(KJV)**

You have heard the saying "Garbage in – Garbage out"; I believe that to be a truth like no other. If we are always letting the bad stuff into our lives, our minds and our circumstances, how can we ever hope to have a positive outlook? For me, I needed to take a step back and look at what I was allowing in my mind and in my life. After putting my focus on Philippians 4:8 I started looking at everything differently. I decided right then and there that I was going to be a "Whatsoever Gal". I would look at the things I talked about, watched, listened to, admired and did. Then I would ask myself the following questions:

1. Is this true?
2. Is this something decent?
3. Is doing this the right thing?
4. Is this innocent and sweet?
5. Is this something to be proud of?
6. Is what I am doing, watching or speaking about good or worthy of praise?

Boy, did that change my outlook and my attitude! Since I had a lot of limitations, I was unable to do much at all. I ended up watching quite a few movies and the television was almost always on. At first my vision was affected and I really could not see to watch, but it was still on in the background. You may think that would not matter and say it was just background noise, but I can honestly say that it did matter. My husband is a big news fan and had the news on a lot. As we all know, the news is not usually reporting good, noble or praiseworthy things. When it was on, whether or not I was actively listening, it was loading garbage in my mind and my heart. Report after report of bad news, devastation and lawlessness was making me miserable and encouraging a negative attitude. I could feel the negativity and the anxiety welling up inside of my heart as I took it in.

Realizing how hearing all of these bad things was changing my outlook, affecting my peace and stealing my joy, I decided to limit what I was putting in my mind through what was on TV. I cannot tell you how my thoughts, dreams and outlook started to change. I even limited my time on Facebook and focused on happy posts and on encouraging others. What a transformation!

I decided to limit my television selections. My friends really got a chuckle out of this, and I have taken quite a bit of ribbing, because the only channel I would allow on around me was Hallmark. It had clean, uplifting, and good movies that touched my heart in a good way. That was something I needed during that season of my life, and to this day I truly appreciate the sweet selection of stories. I am no longer stuck to where I am seeing so much television, but when I do, I still weigh it against the verse in Philippians 4:8.

When I consider how important it is to focus on these things and to have a good attitude, I am reminded of the story of Jonah and how his bad attitude got him into trouble in a BIG way. You see, Jonah was a prophet and God asked him to go to a horrible city to tell them they needed to change. Let's look at his negative response…

Jonah 1:1-3 (NIV)

> *The word of the LORD came to Jonah son of Amittai: "Go to the great city of Nineveh and*

> *preach against it, because its wickedness has come up before me."*
>
> *But Jonah ran away from the LORD and headed for Tarshish. He went down to Joppa, where he found a ship bound for that port. After paying the fare, he went aboard and sailed for Tarshish to flee from the LORD.*

You see, Jonah didn't want to go where God asked him to go. He was afraid and allowed his negative attitude to place him in a panic and make him run in the opposite direction. Did he really think it was possible to run from the Lord? As the story goes on in Jonah 1 we know that while he was on the ship he was escaping in, God sent a huge storm. The men on board became scared and Jonah told them that it was his fault as he was running from the Lord.

Jonah told the men they should throw him overboard and the storm would calm. After some discussion and attempts to head back, they did exactly as he instructed. As Jonah was thrown into the stormy waters, he was swallowed up by a really big fish and HE SURVIVED! Wow, even Jonah knew that the Lord's hand was on him. He had a job to do, and God was showing him how important it is to not only do what he was being called to do, but to trust Him to help get him through even the things that seemed uncertain or impossible. Jonah was in the belly of the fish for 3 entire days; while he was there, he prayed and cried out to the Lord. He confessed everything that had happened and in the end of his prayer he commits to doing what God asked of him in the first place.

Jonah 2:9 (NIV)

> *But I, with shouts of grateful praise will sacrifice to you. What I have vowed I will make good. I will say, 'Salvation comes from the LORD.*

After the 3 days, God had the fish spit Jonah onto dry land. He was obedient and went to Nineveh and told the people of their wicked ways. To Jonah's disappointment, when the Ninevites repented, God showed them mercy. Even after Jonah came around and did what God asked him to do, he still seemed to have a negative outlook. Perhaps he could not look at how the Lord was working in the lives of the people of Nineveh to change their hearts. Perhaps (like we all do), he was hanging onto the past, remembering what the people of Ninevah had done to the Israelites. Sometimes it is hard to let go of past hurts, or situations, and that affects how we deal with our current circumstances. Was that Jonah's problem?

Could he not see how many awesome things the Lord brought him through to speak truth to those in the city? Was he not moved at all by their repentance? Do I ever witness the wonderful works of God around me and still refuse to be in awe and excitement for all He does? When we are called to do something, or we have to endure a trial, are we facing it with confidence and a positive attitude?

Sometimes, just like Jonah, I have gone the wrong way and focused on the negative instead of trusting God. Throughout my surgery and recovery, and my life for that matter, I have learned that a positive attitude is not just what I need, it is something I HAVE to have. From the bottom of my heart, I want to be that "WHATSOEVER GAL" from Philippians 4:8. I cannot do that unless I also strive to follow God's word in Philippians 2:5.

> **Your attitude should be the same as that of Christ Jesus... Philippians 2:5 (NIV)**

Prayer for a negative attitude...

> *Dear Heavenly Father, thank you for Your Word that we can use as a guidebook for our lives! Today I choose to be a "WHATSOEVER GAL" and will measure all that I think, say or do according to your word in*

Philippians 4:8. I ask you to guard my heart and my attitude as I go through each day and focus on the things of you.

Good things!

Praiseworthy things!

Truthful things!

Thank you Lord for your example and guidance on how to live a positive, joy-filled life.

DIAGNOSIS: BEING NEGATIVE

SYMPTOMS: Withdrawal, Apathy, Poor Outlook, Lack of Energy, Jealousy, Anger, Meanness, General Malaise (Icky feeling)

TREATMENT: To overcome a negative attitude, concentrate on the good things all around you and NOT everything that is going wrong. Do NOT compare yourself to others and their situation. It is also imperative to consistently remind yourself of who you serve.

PRESCRIPTION: Be a WHATSOEVER GAL or GUY, focusing on Philippians 4:8. Speak life out loud over your situation. APPLY GENEROUSLY TO EYES to increase focus: concentrating on the good in things. Taking in good thoughts and encouraging scriptures regularly, you will remember who you are as a child of God and notice the SONSHINE that is all around you.

SIDE EFFECTS: May increase your ability to look on the bright side of every situation. USE WITH CARE as you develop your Christ-like attitude and apply it to your life.

CHECKUP

1. Have you been experiencing a negative attitude? Why?

2. How can you let Philippians 4:8 help you get through a tough situation?

3. Is what you are doing, watching or speaking good or worthy of praise?

4. What are you focusing on when times get tough?

5. What kind of negative things in your life are keeping you from seeing the Good in your situation, or your life?

6. What steps can you take to change your attitude toward your circumstances?

7. Do you think your circumstances will improve as you change your attitude?

WORDS OF ENCOURAGEMENT: NO MORE NEGATIVE ATTITUDE!

WHEN YOU ARE NEGATIVE ABOUT YOUR SITUATION... KEEP YOUR FOCUS!

Do not let any unwholesome talk come out of your mouths, but only what is helpful for building others up according to their needs, that it may benefit those who listen. Ephesians 4:29 (NIV)

But seek first his kingdom and his righteousness, and all these things will be given to you as well. Matthew 6:33 (NIV)

So we say with confidence, "The Lord is my helper; I will not be afraid. What can mere mortals do to me?" Hebrews 13:6 (NIV)

WHEN YOU ARE FEELING NEGATIVE... BE CONFIDENT IN CHRIST!

And we know that in all things God works for the good of those who love him, who have been called according to his purpose. Romans 8:28 (NIV)

For I am confident of this very thing, that He who began a good work in you will perfect it until the day of Christ Jesus. (NIV)

"Have I not commanded you? Be strong and courageous! Do not tremble or be dismayed, for the LORD your God is with you wherever you go." (NIV)

WHEN YOU HAVE A BAD ATTITUDE... LOOK TO JESUS!

The LORD'S lovingkindnesses indeed never cease, For His compassions never fail. They are new every morning; Great is Your faithfulness. Lamentations 3:22-23 (NIV)

...and being fully assured that what God had promised, He was able also to perform. Romans 4:21 (NIV)

If we are faithless, He remains faithful, for He cannot deny Himself. 2 Timothy 2:13(NIV)

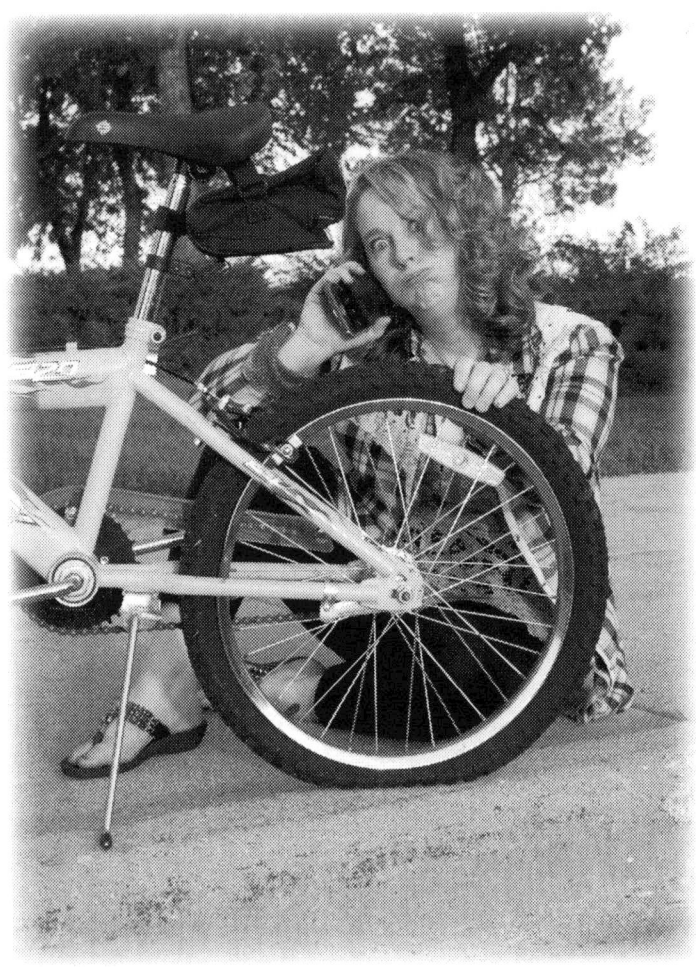

A Negative Attitude is like a flat tire... You can't go anywhere until you change it. (Author Unknown)

LESSON FOUR

DON'T **I**SOLATE YOURSELF

"I am so lonely!" Those are words that my husband heard come out of my mouth more often than I care to admit over the past few years. It is so hard to admit something like that, and even harder to share.

I come from a long line of talkers. I have always been an outspoken, talkative person and my love language is definitely time and communication. I could sit and talk with friends and family, or strangers for that matter, for hours on end. In fact, many years ago, as my husband and I were traveling on our honeymoon, I was sitting out on the deck at the hotel near the pool. He came to join me and saw that I was in deep conversation with about 4 other people. Being the sweet guy he is, he just joined right in on the conversation without hesitation.

After we had visited for over an hour, we parted ways with hugs, saying it was great to see each other and looked forward to meeting again. About an hour later, my husband said to me "It was really great meeting your friends, where do you know them from?" I turned to him and said, "I didn't know them, I just met them tonight." He laughed so hard, because, with the depth of our conversation and our sweet goodbyes, he thought they were practically family. That has happened so many times over the years and it is just as true today as it was years ago. I love people... getting to know them, encouraging them, and just spending time with them. I am so blessed by that.

During my recovery, I enjoyed so many precious times with visitors, especially in the first few months. People all around me were so faithful to come and sit with me and help in my care. I was very thankful for that. As time went on and I gained a little more independence, daily cares were not needed like they were before, and I was spending more and more time by myself. My family would come home from school and work and go about their business. The world was going on around me and I was just kind of stuck where I was at.

Being by myself for most of the day without a lot to do began to take its toll on me and I felt so alone. I know that loneliness is something that affects all of us at one time or another. I tried to just keep my mind occupied, but since I was physically unable to do a lot, talking with people was all I had. I had a difficult time letting people know that. It can be hard when you feel isolated from so many things, and that isolation can happen in different ways. Sometimes people are lonely because they isolate themselves, but I was isolated by my circumstances.

Living in a house with all boys doesn't give me a lot of chances to be chatty either. At this particular time, I had been very lonesome. I was still somewhat bedridden and the only time I got to really sit and talk with anyone was if someone called or stopped by.

Maybe you have been there? As I pointed out in the beginning of this book, it was not always easy for me to share things that show vulnerability, and when I tried to express my loneliness to friends. I got responses anywhere from tears to flowers. It was a very hard season, and that loneliness created a kind of depression that was starting to hinder my recovery. At one point, I actually carried on a 30-minute phone call with a sales lady, just because I needed to talk.

It began on an afternoon when I was just sitting there feeling kind of sorry for myself and very alone. I had spoken with my mother earlier that day and she had said that she talked with my aunt from Kentucky. My mom said that she had asked about me and how I was doing. When my phone rang and my caller ID said it was a Kentucky call, I was kind of excited and thought it just might be her on the other end of the line. Sure enough, I answer, and the lady said her name and it even sounded just like my aunt's name. Either it wasn't a great connection, or I was just desperate to talk to someone and I assumed it was her. Nonetheless I just started talking and talking and talking to her... I told her everything that had been going on in my life for the last few weeks and even more. I did think it was kind of funny every time she asked me about my windows, but that really didn't seem too odd given that we had our front window break when my husband was trying to find time, between work and caring for me, to change out our storm windows. I just assumed that was what she was referring to each time she asked. I simply thought my mother had probably told her about our broken front window.

As the conversation continued and I just talked and talked and poured out my heart like I hadn't spoken with anyone for ages, the lady was very quiet. In fact, about 25 to 35 minutes had passed. Finally, I had to breathe and the lady quickly got a sentence in saying "You know I have really enjoyed chatting with you, but I don't think I am who you think I am." My reply then, was "Who are you?" I was finally quiet long enough to listen as she said "I am so and so from a window company out of Kentucky and we would like to send someone over from our Madison office to give you an estimate on new windows." Well, bless her heart, I sure hope she was being paid by the minute. I could not believe I had been pouring out my heart to a complete stranger. Needless to say, we did not need any new windows, but I did learn a lesson.

Lesson Learned: It is ok to be vulnerable. When we are feeling lonely or isolated, we don't have to look for someone to share with. We can pour our hearts out to God. He will always listen (and NEVER try to sell us any windows). We can ask Him to bring someone into our lives that will brighten our day, lift our spirits and point us to him. We can share how we feel with those around us and not feel uncomfortable or odd. He has shown me that over and over again, throughout my recovery.

Another lonely time I experienced while I was in the hospital really showed me how much the Lord cares about my situation. He not only heard my plea, but answered my prayer for someone to talk to me. He sent someone to encourage me and pray for me within minutes of my cries to Him. What a mighty and loving God we serve!

Here is my story...

The hospital room was so quiet. It was an eerie and uncomfortable silence that made my heart feel extremely heavy and my mind was preoccupied with overwhelming thoughts of loneliness. I was sitting in the wheelchair, just looking ahead at things that almost seemed unrecognizable. My vision was still blurry after the surgery and my abilities were limited. The boredom blues really started to set in. I had been in the hospital for some time, but this was my very first day being all alone. Prior to this, my family and friends had always been by my side, talking with me and keeping me company. The time had come for my kids to go back to school, my parents to get back home, and my husband to go back to work. I was in a safe place for recovery, but my mind began to wander into a world of loneliness that felt so heavy on my heart.

Frankly, I was feeling rather sorry for myself and just did not know what to do. I started crying out to the Lord, telling Him how lonely I was and how helpless I felt, as if He didn't know. Through my tears I pled with him to bring someone to talk to me, to sit with me, or just to take a moment to brighten my day. I am not sure of the time frame, but it honestly felt like not even a moment went by after I had petitioned the Lord for a friend. In His graciousness, my Heavenly Father answered my cries for help. He knew my circumstances and as I lifted my head I saw the door to my room open, There was a beautiful smiling face, clear as a bell. It was not someone I expected to see, I had not seen her in some time, so it was a wonderful gift.

You see, this friend had been struggling for years with a recurrence of cancer and was just undergoing another scan to check on the progress of her treatments. With all that was surely weighing on her mind, I could not believe that she came to lift my spirits. What a blessing that was!

God knew exactly what I needed, just when I needed it. He was there for me and brought someone into my life at that moment, to help me through my day. Someone who surely understood my circumstance. We laughed together and she prayed for me and allowed me to pray for her. I am so thankful for our time together. She wasn't there long, but she was there when I needed her, and her beautiful smile and encouraging spirit touched my heart that was feeling so sad. I just love how the Lord works in our lives. He truly wants more for us than we can even imagine. As a parent, we understand the love we have for our children and that we would do just about anything to keep them happy. I am so thankful that my Heavenly Father feels that way toward each and every one of His children as well.

In God's Word we can look to Jeremiah to see an example of loneliness. Jeremiah had been called to be a prophet of God before he was even born.

> *"Before I formed you in the womb I knew you, before you were born I set you apart; I appointed you as a prophet to the nations." Jeremiah 1:5 (NIV)*

What was he called to do? Jeremiah was called to tell the people of Israel that they needed to repent from their wicked ways and turn back to God. That was certainly easier said than done. Jeremiah preached for decades, and still they would not listen. To make things worse, he was all alone in his message and circumstances. He did not get to marry and had no friends or family around for support. It was a very lonely life.

That lonely life made Jeremiah get so overwhelmed at times that he would become very depressed and that left him at times questioning God's plans and his own calling.

> *Why is my pain unending and my wound grievous and incurable? You are to me like a deceptive brook, like a spring that fails. Jeremiah 15:18 (NIV)*

He felt like he was all alone and that he wasn't even making a difference. In verse 19, God is telling him to repent of his "bad attitude" and then He will restore him and can use him as He had planned all along.

> *Therefore this is what the LORD says: "If you repent, I will restore you that you may serve me; if you utter worthy, not worthless, words, you will be my spokesman. Let this people turn to you, but you must not turn to them... Jeremiah 15:19 (NIV)*

The Lord reminded Jeremiah who he was and what he was being called to do. You see, when Jeremiah would concentrate on himself and his loneliness, he would lose focus on God's plan for his life. God knew Jeremiah was lonely, but Jeremiah forgot that God was always with him, giving him words to say and being his constant companion.

In the same way, we can lose sight of the bigger picture and become totally overwhelmed with our circumstances. In those moments, we tend to isolate ourselves even more, and sometimes we turn our backs on God. We may even be thinking… if He really loved us, He would never allow us to go through such a hard time. Jeremiah shows us that even someone who has such a high calling as a prophet can go through times of loneliness and even become depressed as he goes about the Lord's business. We can rejoice in the fact that no matter what we are going through, or how discouraged we feel, God is always with us. Just like Jeremiah, He knew us before we were born and has BIG plans for our lives. We need to remember the verse that we have mentioned in several of the previous chapters. Jeremiah 29:11 reminds us of the plans for our future and what God says about each of us… I feel it deserves repeating in this chapter.

> *For I know the plans I have for you," declares the LORD, "plans to prosper you and not to harm you, plans to give you hope and a future. Jeremiah 29:11(NIV)*

Prayer for a lonely heart…

> *Dear Heavenly Father, thank you for Your promise to always stay right beside us no matter what we are going through. I give you my loneliness and today I choose to give you my whole self and come to you as my comfort and friend. I ask you to touch my heart as I live each day for you. When I feel lonely, I know you will help me…*

> *Feel loved!*

> *Share love!*

Accept love!

Thank you Lord for your love and touch on my life so that I will live and celebrate the plans that you have for me.

DIAGNOSIS: LONELINESS

SYMPTOMS: Withdrawal, Feelings of Being All Alone, Sadness, Isolation, Lack of Energy, Depression, General Malaise (Icky feeling)

TREATMENT: To overcome loneliness, remember who you are as a Child of God and that He is always right beside you. Pray often. Find a good Christian fellowship to worship with. Surround yourself with encouraging people. Take some time to spend with friends and family. Do not spend a lot of time thinking of, or dwelling on, things you cannot change in your life, but rather ask God to help you through them.

PRESCRIPTION: Take some time to dig deep into the Word of God. Go visit with or invite a friend to go out for coffee or lunch. Go somewhere you enjoy. Think about doing something for someone else.

SIDE EFFECTS: May increase feelings of contentment. When taken as directed, you will see your focus move away from yourself and your problems and onto what the Lord has planned for you.

<u>CHECKUP</u>

1. Have you been experiencing a time of loneliness? Why?

2. Do you ever feel like you are stuck in life or in your circumstance?

3. When you feel lonely, what do you do?

4. Do you have someone to talk to when you are feeling alone?

5. Are you spending time with the Lord every day?

6. What can you do to help yourself when you are having a hard time?

7. Are there ways that you can get involved in church activities or Bible studies?

WORDS OF ENCOURAGEMENT: OVERCOMING LONELINESS!

WHEN YOU ARE FEELING LONELY... TURN TO GOD!

Turn to me and be gracious to me, for I am lonely and afflicted. Psalm 25:16 (NIV)

But let all who take refuge in you rejoice; let them ever sing for joy, and spread your protection over them, that those who love your name may exult in you. Psalm 5:11 (NIV)

Trust in him at all times, O people; pour out your heart before him; God is a refuge for us. Psalm 62:8 *(NIV)*

Commit your way to the LORD; trust in him, and he will do this. Psalm 37:5 (NIV)

WHEN YOU ARE DISTRESSED... LET GOD COMFORT YOU!

He heals the brokenhearted and binds up their wounds. Psalm 147:3 (NIV)

Cast all your anxiety on him because he cares for you. 1 Peter 5:7 (NIV)

Peace I leave with you; my peace I give you. I do not give to you as the world gives. Do not let your hearts be troubled and do not be afraid. *John 14:27* (NIV)

WHEN YOU ARE UNHAPPY... BE FILLED WITH JOY!

Consider it pure joy, my brothers and sisters, whenever you face trials of many kinds, because you know that the testing of your faith produces perseverance. James 1:2-3 (NIV)

May the God of hope fill you with all joy and peace as you trust in him, so that you may overflow with hope by the power of the Holy Spirit. Romans 15:13 (NIV)

Your love has given me great joy and encouragement, because you, brother, have refreshed the hearts of the Lord's people. Philemon 1:7 (NIV)

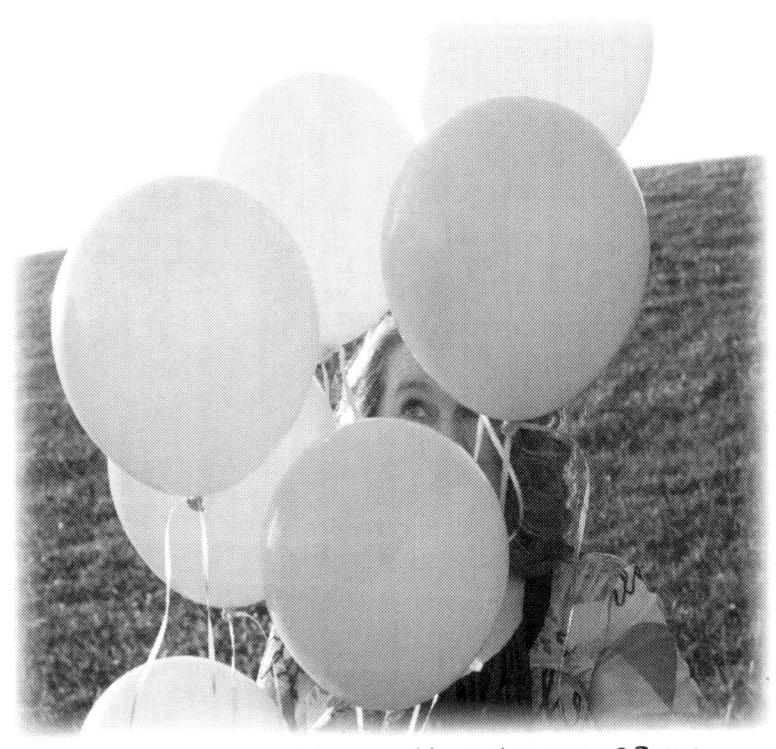

Look past your problems and into the eyes of Jesus...

LESSON FIVE

DON'T BE <u>C</u>RABBY
OR <u>C</u>OMPLAIN

The **MOST** important lesson I learned throughout my ordeal really draws together all of the others in the previous chapters of **DON'T PANIC**. (Don't <u>P</u>lant Seeds of Doubt, Don't Be <u>A</u>nxious, Don't Be <u>N</u>egative, Don't <u>I</u>solate Yourself, and now, Don't Be <u>C</u>rabby or <u>C</u>omplain).

I learned this most important lesson the day that I realized how important it is to have a cheerful heart, even during the worst of circumstances. Being cheerful can really be a hard thing to accomplish when you are overwhelmed by your situation, like I had been. The Lord really had to show me how to get through each and every day and how not to complain or be crabby, even when I wanted to. I am so thankful for His message to us in Proverbs 17:22. It really changed my whole outlook and altered my focus during this battle with brain surgery and recovery.

> *A cheerful heart is good medicine; but a crushed*
> *spirit dries up the bones. Proverbs 17:22 (NIV)*

You might say like I did, "Lord, how in the world am I supposed to have a cheerful heart when I am going through such a hard time?" After I read this verse over and over again, I pictured the Lord saying "Oh Jeaunetta, I am so glad you asked… If you have a cheerful heart, then you will stop looking at yourself and start to look ahead and look up for help with your situation. If you do not have a cheerful heart and your spirit is broken, there will be nothing to fight with to get through this trial, no matter what it is." I realized that the Lord had reminded me through this verse just how much I needed that foundation of JOY that I spoke of earlier. We ALL need it!

Sometimes, we allow our circumstances to dictate our opinions and outlook. If we are enduring a difficult time, then the last thing we should do is focus on the problem itself. That focus can make us see only the bad in our situation. Then that can make us angry or bitter, and certainly makes us crabby.

I really don't like to complain, but I do know that complaining is part of human nature. It seems to come so easy. Perhaps we complain because we don't like something, we don't want to do something, or just don't like what is happening to us. We live in an age where, if something is irritating us, we like to let people know about it. Then, when our situation does not change the way we want it to or, it gets worse… We complain about it and get crabbier and crabbier.

Have you ever been around someone who complains all of the time? They are miserable. After you listen to it over and over, it makes you miserable too. They are just plain CRABBY and it seems that their only purpose in life is to complain about everything. You feel like there is nothing you can do or say to improve their outlook, and pretty soon you are sucked into the vortex of grumbling. It is very sad, and hard to escape from. That complaining spirit can especially be detrimental to you when you face a trial or impossible circumstance. I know for me, it seemed that as I allowed something small to get me in a funk, every little thing that happened just made my attitude snowball. When that would happen, I would be miserable and make everyone around me, miserable too.

In the hospital rehab program, I met so many people. Some were in for just a short time, while others were there for an extended stay, like me. The circumstances were different for all of us and yet quite similar. From stroke recovery and brain tumors to car crashes with traumatic brain injuries, we all had one thing in common - we were there to heal.

The outlook and attitude of each individual was as different as the circumstances. Some were strong and quiet, some talked a lot, and some were very angry about their situation. It was definitely a hard road for everyone there. However, there was one thing that I noticed immediately: the recovery process of those who had a positive outlook. It was very noticeable, and I could tell that it was something that affected everything they did with each step forward. Don't get me wrong, going through difficult circumstances is tremendously hard and may feel nearly impossible, causing an influx of negative emotions. Those emotions can overcome you and fill your mind with bad images, bad ideas and a very scary outlook. Who wouldn't complain? We all have moments, but when those moments turn into hours and days and we cannot get back to a positive train of thought, let me tell you what can happen...

An attitude of crabbiness and complaining can affect any and all of the following when you are going through a tough time:

- Your hope
- Your endurance
- Your outlook
- Your recovery
- Your healing
- Your life

*Your **hope*** is affected when you are complaining because you are always looking to the dark side of any situation. If you are always looking down, you will never be able to see what is ahead. God gives us an eternal hope that can help us through any and every situation. Today may look dark, but eternity is bright.

*Your **endurance*** is lowered because you have invested all of your energy into speaking negatively about your situation. God says He will help us to run the race set before us and never leave us or forsake us. Let the Lord energize your spirit with His power.

*Your **outlook*** is skewed because you are looking at and concentrating on the bad in your situation. You know it is hard to see any good or to look ahead when you are always looking back. God tells us to keep our eyes on Him and He will show us the way He has set for us. Let the Lord open your eyes to all He has in store for you!

*Your **recovery*** is hindered because attitude is everything when you are trying to heal from a sickness, or even a bad situation. God will strengthen you to get through difficult times. You need not worry or fear. Turn to the Lord and give Him everything that is dragging you down today.

*Your **healing*** is unavailable because all of your faith is swept up in the focus on what's not right in your situation. God's Word says without faith it's impossible to please Him. He says believe and you will be healed. Let the Lord in and trust Him with your entire situation.

*Your **life*** is affected because you can't be happy or fruitful when you are constantly tearing down everything that could build you up, nor, when you are constantly planting seeds of doubt within yourself or your situation. God says that we are His children and co-heirs with Jesus. Remember who you belong to and start treating yourself as a child of the King.

As I got to know some of the people that were straining and struggling during the recovery process, just like me, I began to appreciate every one of them. I would admire them and acknowledge the difficulty of what they were each going through. One of the best examples that I can think of that shows how a cheerful heart really is good medicine happened during a simple Occupational Therapy group.

There we were in the large group OT therapy room. It was just me, Harold and Bernadette in the room with our therapists. We were working on things that most would consider easy, everyday tasks. Harold had been in an accident and his rehab that day was working on counting and putting some coins in a bank. Even though it was a struggle, he was doing very well. Bernadette was a stroke survivor and she was working on the everyday task of folding towels and washcloths; she really did a good job. This day was especially difficult for me, as I was trying to tie a shoe. At first glance, I shrugged my shoulders and thought… I can do this, how hard can it be? After all, I have been tying my shoes since I was five years old. As they wheeled me in to my work table, I see a giant shoe with laces right in front of me. I start looking at the others as they struggle through their tasks, but are ultimately successful. With a nod of the therapist's head, I reach out to start to tie.

As my hands got to the laces with great anticipation, I realized something very significant… **I HAD NO IDEA** what I was doing. My mind was blank, I moved the laces around a little, trying so hard to remember; but nothing. It wasn't even something I could fake. As I kept trying to remember, I became quite stressed. My hands were shaking more than they were before and finally the therapist asked me if I could remember how to do it. My face at that moment must have looked twisted and funny as Harold began to crack up and says out loud, "She can't tie her shoe". Then Bernadette joins in, laughing like crazy. I looked up and saw a funny moment and said to Harold "What are you guys laughing at? You can't count quarters and she can't fold a washcloth." That was it, the therapists had lost all control. We all giggled and giggled at our circumstances that day, and boy did that feel good. That joy and laughter in the midst of such defeat gave us that push that we needed to move on and keep trying. From that moment on, we had smiles on our faces and joy in our hearts as we came together to work on our recovery.

When I consider how important it is to focus on cheerful things and to have a good attitude, even in the worst of times, I am reminded of the Israelites as they were heading to the promised land. As we look at the story of Moses and the deliverance of God's people, we see celebration and read the beautiful song praising God for giving them strength and helping them out of an impossible situation. In the beginning of Exodus, the children of Israel had just seen how God had parted the sea to make way for their escape. The beginning verses are my favorite, and I can even remember singing them in church as a child.

> *Then Moses and the Israelites sang this song to the LORD: "I will sing to the LORD, for he is highly exalted. Both horse and driver he has hurled into the sea."*
>
> *The LORD is my strength and my defense; he has become my salvation.*
>
> *He is my God, and I will praise him, my father's God, and I will exalt him. Exodus 15:1-2 (NIV)*

I find it interesting that it did not take long for them to go from praising to complaining as soon as times got tough. Here is what happened just a few short verses later…

> *Then Moses led Israel from the Red Sea and they went into the Desert of Shur. For three days they traveled in the desert without finding water. When they came to Marah, they could not drink its water because it was bitter. (That is why the place is called Marah.) So the people grumbled against Moses, saying, "What are we to drink?" Exodus 15:22-24 (NIV)*

The children of Israel had just witnessed this AMAZING miracle in the parting of the Red Sea, and yet just a few days later they are complaining about their situation and doubting that God will take care of their needs. WOW! That seems ridiculous, but it made me start to think… Is that something I have done when things go wrong? Do I rejoice in something good that the Lord has done in my life and then, moments later, become nervous and worried that things are not going the way I want? Have I done that throughout my recovery?

When we go through trials and come out on the other side of them, we can usually look back and see how the Lord has worked on us, in us, and through us. Sometimes, I must admit, that like the Israelites, I have not remembered that He has got it covered. Now, I can say that through my recent experiences, I have learned that the most important thing that I can do, and the only thing I CAN control, is my attitude. I want it to be a positive one that looks for the good in everything. Once again, I need to strive to be a "Whatsoever gal" who is trying to to keep a positive attitude even in the worst of circumstances.

Prayer for a complaining heart…

> *Dear Heavenly Father, thank you for being the Lord of all good things! Today I choose to focus on all that you give me, and ask for forgiveness for the times when I have complained about my circumstances. I will stand on all that you do to touch my heart during difficult situations.*
>
> *I stand on peace!*
>
> *I stand on hope!*
>
> *I stand on love!*
>
> *Thank you for pointing me in the right direction as I stand on Your Word at all times.*

DIAGNOSIS: WAY TOO CRABBY

SYMPTOMS: Negative, Irritable, Poor Outlook, Lack of Energy, Jealousy, Anger, Spitefulness, Self-Centered, General Malaise (Icky feeling)

TREATMENT: To overcome Crabbiness and a Complaining attitude, try to find a bright spot about your circumstance. Do NOT Complain about your situation constantly. Try listing 2 good things that are happening with every bad thing you see.

PRESCRIPTION: Go to the Lord daily and ask Him to restore Joy to your life and over your situation. Fill yourself full of the promises we find in scriptures. Focus on your words and only release the ones that are uplifting and beneficial to you and your recovery. Take some quality time to rejuvenate and refresh your attitude.

SIDE EFFECTS: You may develop a greater passion for your recovery in both your body and your mind. Your circumstance and outlook may appear brighter with each and every day. Consistent intake of God's promises may remove unwanted irritants.

CHECKUP

1. Have you noticed that you have been really crabby lately? Why?

2. How have you allowed it to affect yourself and those around you?

3. Do you spend more time complaining about your situation than you do in recovery?

4. What is one good thing that you can focus on right now?

5. What can you do to focus on the POSITIVE in your circumstance?

6. Do you think that complaining about or being crabby about things is affecting you in a negative way?

7. List a few things that you are willing to do to change how you are reacting to your situation...

WORDS OF ENCOURAGEMENT: NO MORE COMPLAINING!

WHEN YOU ARE COMPLAINING ABOUT YOUR SITUATION... STOP NOW!

Do everything without grumbling... Philippians 2:14 (NIV)

"But one thing I do: Forgetting what is behind and straining toward what is ahead, I press on toward the goal to win the prize for which God has called me heavenward in Christ Jesus" Philippians 3:13-14 (NIV)

"Let no unwholesome word proceed from your mouth, but only such a word as is good for edification according to the need of the moment, so that it will give grace to those who hear." Ephesians 4:29 (NIV)

WHEN YOU ARE FEELING CRABBY... FOCUS ON THE GOODNESS OF GOD!

Teach me to do Your will, For You are my God; Let Your good Spirit lead me on level ground. Psalm 143:10 (NIV)

Sovereign LORD, you are God! Your covenant is trustworthy, and you have promised these good things to your servant. Samuel 7:28 (NIV)

Do not conform to the pattern of this world, but be transformed by the renewing of your mind. Then you will be able to test and approve what God's will is—his good, pleasing and perfect will. Romans 12:2 (NIV)

WHEN YOU ARE DOWN AND DEPRESSED... LOOK FOR GOOD!

"I am leaving you with a gift - peace of mind and heart. And the peace I give is a gift the world cannot give. So don't be troubled or afraid." John 14:27 (NIV)

"And this same God who takes care of me will supply all your needs from his glorious riches, which have been given to us in Christ Jesus." Philippians 4:19 (NIV)

"Come to me, all you who are weary and burdened, and I will give you rest. Take my yoke upon you and learn from me, for I am gentle and humble in heart, and you will find rest for your souls." Matthew 11:28-29. (NIV)

DON'T PANIC REVIEW

Don't **P**lant Seeds of Doubt!

Don't be **A**nxious!

Don't be **N**egative!

Don't **I**solate Yourself!

Don't **C**omplain!

THE PRESCRIPTION FOR A HEALTHY & HAPPY LIFE

As I was going through my recovery, I would sometimes think to myself… "Why me?" Why would the Lord allow me to go through such a hard time? Did He know how miserable I was? I knew perfectly well that the answer to that question was very clear… Why not me? Why would I even think that I would be exempt from the troubles of this world? Sometimes in our human nature and self-centered thought process, we start to expect preferential treatment as Christians. When we don't get that treatment we believe we should get, we might even become bitter or angry with God or actually blame Him for our circumstances.

Years ago, I can remember a Christian friend, who was experiencing a bad week, saying to me "I just don't know why God is doing this to me?" I told her we have all had times where we have questioned our circumstances and asked God why He allows bad things to happen, but it is important to remember that God doesn't cause any of it. John 10:10 (KJV) reminds us who is to blame for our troubles:

> **The thief cometh not, but for to steal, and to kill, and to destroy: I am come that they might have life, and that they might have it more abundantly.**
> **John 10:10 (KJV)**

He wants us to experience good things and to live an abundant life. Bad things happen because we live in a sinful world, not because God wants to hurt us or see us miserable. He does not **WANT** us to experience sickness, pain or hurt of any kind, but when we do, we can count on this… He is right there to be our protector, our comforter and our shield. If it weren't for Him, things would be so much worse. Maybe, like so many of us, you are asking why God doesn't spare you from horrible circumstances as His child. We may even think it is unfair when we go through tough times, but the truth is that God tells us in His Word (Matthew 5:45) that bad things happen to everyone, the righteous and unrighteous.

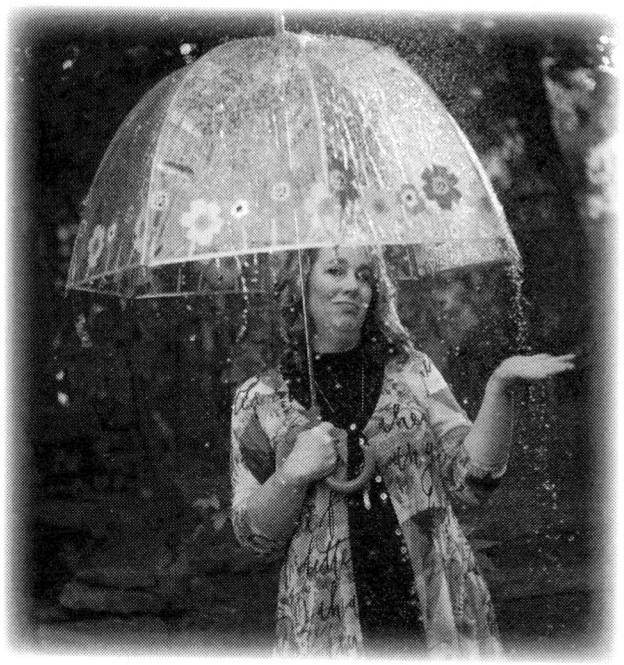

...that you may be children of your Father in heaven. He causes his sun to rise on the evil and the good, and sends rain on the righteous and the unrighteous. Matthew 5:45 (NIV)

I have had so many people ask me why I am not angry about my circumstances with my health. I don't think it is as simple as that question. At times I have been very burdened by my circumstances, but as I think about what I have gone through, my thoughts turn to others that have suffered even greater pain and troubles. I think about my friends who have lost children, who I am sure have expressed anger and frustration about their situation. I think about my mother, sister-in-law, niece, and the many friends who have gone through horrible cancer treatments, or my friends who are stuck in dead end jobs or horrible relationships. Once again, I must point myself in the direction of the truth, and the truth is, we all have different paths to travel and sometimes the way seems dark, rocky and almost impassable. It is never an easy and smooth sailing road for anyone, even when it seems like it is. No matter where you are in your journey, I promise you the ride will be much smoother when God is right beside you. When we get angry with God or blame Him for every bad circumstance in our lives, we are separating ourselves from the only help (and hope for that matter) that we have available as we travel down the rocky road of life.

As I look back on some of the lessons I have learned throughout my journey, I see that I was the one who needed to change my attitude, my outlook, my thought process, my focus and my associations with others. I was the one that was constantly changing according to my circumstance. The Lord would always stay the same. That was a hard swallow, because I must say that change can be hard, or at least I know it has been for me. When my body hurts or it doesn't work the way I want or need it to, and when I struggle to do the simplest tasks, it is frustrating and can be very discouraging, making it very easy to give up or give in.

How was I going to train my brain to respond differently and change my way of dealing with, or reacting to, my struggles. I did not want to live defeated. I wanted to live in victory and I knew it was possible. I knew that was what the Lord had for me, and it is what He has for all of His children. So what would I do? I decided that I was going to look at it from the perspective of a patient who is in dire need of an appointment with the GREAT PHYSICIAN!

Why didn't I think about that before? If there is anything that I have learned throughout my diagnosis, treatment and recovery, it is that I always need to rely on someone who knows more about my circumstance than I do. In the DON'T PANIC lessons, I learned how to get through different aspects of treatment and recovery with the Lord's Help, but what else can I do to keep me living victoriously throughout my recovery and my life?

I have certainly been to many, many Doctor visits, and there is one thing the Dr. does that helps us to keep moving in the best direction for recovery so we can live a healthy and happy life.

It is a well-known fact that you rarely leave the Doctor's office without a prescription or instructions of some sort. Perhaps it is medication, or some basic instructions to get through whatever is ailing you at the time. It might even be for physical therapy to get you moving a little better. Thinking about those prescriptions or instructions made me start to think that the best and most important thing I can share with each and every one of you who is struggling in one way or another is a Prescription to help you get through a tough time. Let's to take a look at what the Great Physician tells us in His Word.

It doesn't matter what you are dealing with… whether it is your health, or another stressful situation, this prescription will help you get through even the worst of circumstances. Frankly, it is just what the Doctor ordered for a happy and healthy life.

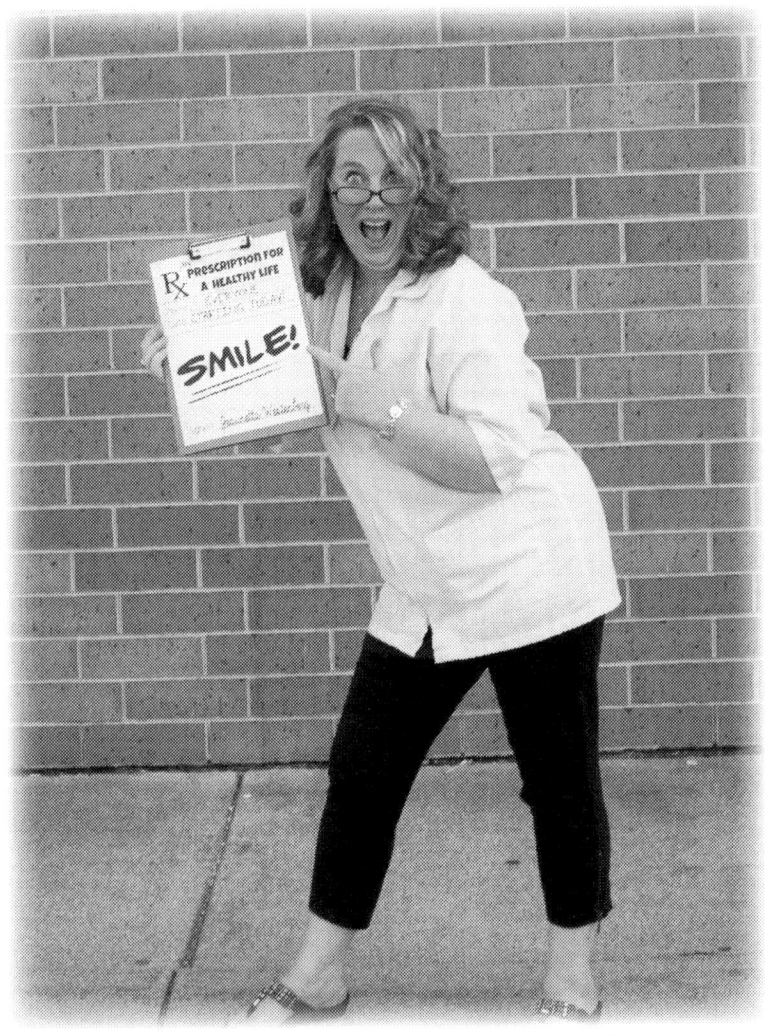

The prescription itself is very simple... S.M.I.L.E.

SCRIPT ONE

SUBMIT OURSELVES TO THE LORD

Trust in the Lord with all your heart, and do not lean on your own understanding, in all your ways acknowledge him & he will make your paths straight. Proverbs 3:5-6 (ESV)

The very first thing we need to do to live a Happy and Healthy life is to SUBMIT OURSELVES TO THE LORD who is our Great Physician. Living a life with an illness or, problems of any kind can be stifling and devastating if we try to handle them on our own. As I discussed earlier… in my circumstances, I wanted to appear as if I always had everything under control, and the "never let them see you sweat" mentality. I cannot believe the amount of time that I wasted carrying my own burdens when the Lord was right there ready to help me.

In the beginning, I was determined to get though my brain surgery kind of like a bull in a china shop. I was just going to do it, get it done and not think about the process or anything else, because the more I thought about it, the harder it was to deal with. I even found myself trying to distract my mind and ignore what I was going through, which caused a lot of unnecessary strife. When someone would ask me how I was doing, I would say really silly things like "I can't complain" or I might even use my Dad's favorite answer… "Better than I deserve." What did those things even mean? I really think they were a diversion tactic so that I wouldn't have to share anything that made me feel vulnerable. I didn't want anyone to know I was weak. In those moments, I was overwhelmed and failed to remember and recognize that when I am weak, God gives me strength. Usually, if I said something like "I can't complain," I would get a small chuckle and a response something like "No one would listen anyway, right?" I think that is also what I thought. How sad is that? Have you ever had someone say that to you? What I really needed was someone to say in those difficult moments was "I know how you feel and I understand it". I did not get those responses because they had no idea that I was struggling, they had no idea I needed encouragement at all. People missed opportunities to be a blessing because I could not share my true feelings.

Now, as I think back, I am also sad and wonder how many opportunities did I miss to share and encourage others who may have been going through something horrible themselves, because I didn't want to appear needy? My entire philosophy has changed as I have learned to deal with difficult circumstances. The fact is that the most important thing we really need to do when we are facing our greatest obstacles in our lives, is to surrender all and just give it to Jesus. I am not going to lie… **IT IS HARD**, but He alone is able to help us carry the load of our burdens and strengthen us as we go to be a light for someone else. He may choose to do that by bringing Godly people into our lives to help us through whatever we are going through, or He may use your struggle to help others. I must say that I have learned so many things in my moments of vulnerability that

I have shared and I have seen the Lord work in mighty ways as I surrendered to Him and then allowed Him to use me to help others.

When I think about our trials, I am reminded of being a child and trying to move something all alone. I would struggle and strain to even budge what I was wanting to move. It seemed like an impossible task, but when my father would see me struggle, he would come over and, with little effort, move the object just where it needed to go. It is the same with our Heavenly Father. When we give everything to Him and stop struggling and straining, He can gently help us move beyond our circumstances. We can look to Him and He will touch our situation and help us to go in the direction He sees best for us.

Sometimes when we are going through a tough time, we don't understand it and we start getting off-track, making life harder and harder. Proverbs 3:5-6 tells us not to lean on our own understanding because we do not see the entire picture. It says that He will make our paths straight as we put all of our trust in Him. Oh, how I want my path straight! I want to Submit my life and everything in it to the Lord and put all of my trust in Him… How about you?

CHECKUP

1. In what ways have you given your circumstances to the Lord?

2. Is there anything happening in your situation that is keeping you from total trust in God?

3. How are you leaning on your own understanding more than leaning on the Lord today?

4. Are you honest with those around you about what you are going through?

5. What steps will you take to give yourself and your circumstances to God if you are not already?

SCRIPT TWO

MAKE THE MOST OF EVERYDAY

Whatever you do, work at it with all your heart, as working for the Lord, not for man since you know that you will receive an inheritance from the Lord as a re-ward. It is the Lord Christ you are serving. Colossians 3:23-24 (NIV)

When sickness and tragedy strike, we can be so devastated that our whole life seems to be under a dark cloud. We barely get by and the days seem to disappear one after another without us seeing any light. I know that is how I felt during certain times of my recovery, and I realized that, during those moments, I really needed to look to the Lord more than ever as my great Physician and Healer. When I would get in a funk and feel like there was no hope for a brighter tomorrow, that is where the Lord would step in and remind me just how precious this life is. I am always amazed that even in the midst of our trials, the Lord shows us how important it is to live life to the fullest. As our Great Physician, God gives us instructions about living and service and the prescription for working at things with all of our heart, serving the Lord in everything we do.

The best part of any prescription is when we start to feel better because we followed the Doctor's instructions. That is exactly what can happen as we do what God tells us to do in His Word.

During my recovery, I certainly had times where I felt bad both physically and emotionally. It was a struggle to accomplish anything. Whatever I would do during those trying times would never be done to the best of my ability. The truth is, I don't think I even cared at that moment. It wasn't until I saw a friend struggling with depression and witnessed her lack of zeal for anything, that I took a closer look at how I was reacting to my struggle with the brain tumor, surgery and the recovery. How was I going to help her, when I had not even been able to help myself? I started to question if I was doing all that I could to accomplish everything that God was calling me to do. And, was I willing to do it as if I was doing it for Him? There it is… No matter where we are within our struggle, we have to **M**AKE THE MOST OF EVERY DAY! It will not be easy as we are trying to just live and get through each day, but we can have victory and make the most of every day by making a conscious decision to work at life as if we are working directly for the Lord. Even if this life is a temp job at best, we need to continually work on our ETERNAL resume. I like to look at it this way and sing this song as I go through some of the hardest days. "This is the day that the Lord has made, I will rejoice and be glad in it." That is something that really changes my outlook on things when I fall into the pit, and it helps me throughout the struggle as my focus goes toward rejoicing and away from myself.

As I turn my focus toward the Lord, I start to remember my purpose, and that is to be an example and tell others about Jesus. Colossians 3:23-24 is the message that I have been sharing. It reminds me that, no matter what I do, I am to be working with all my heart as if working for the Lord, not man.

Again, I need to ask myself… Have I been concentrating on myself and my problems so much so that all I can do is talk about that and live in a miserable funk? Do I make the most of every day, by sharing the gospel message with people I know, or even those I don't?

In the hospital, I can recall everyone telling me that the first thing I did after my surgery, and for a good solid week was ask if my visitors had brought me any chocolate. It was like that was the only thing I had on my mind and it became kind of a joke and, somewhat of a challenge for those who came to see me. After a few weeks, my candy stash was overflowing and we decided I needed to share. I started giving it out by the bagful to those I would visit with or had in therapy groups. It wasn't long before I was known as the "little girl who had chocolate". One day, I was sitting in the doorway of my room in my wheelchair when my friend Bernadette came down the hall walking with her nurse. She quickly waved and pointed me out saying "There's the nice little girl who gives me chocolate". I smiled thinking the nurse would acknowledge my kindness. Then listened to her quick reply and saw her chastising nod my way. She said "Now Bernadette, you know that you are NOT supposed to have sugar!" Bernadette's response was the best... She said "Well, you ONLY LIVE ONCE!" She is so right and that was a great response and so true. We only have this one life, this one opportunity to live, to make the most of every day we are given... What are we doing with it? (For the record, I still didn't want any trouble so I wheeled my chair as fast as I could into my room and didn't come out until their walk was over.)

I now understood why she would hide the candy I gave her in a small box in her closet. She was saving something special to make her day a little tastier when she needed it. My husband always laughs and says that the day after I left the unit, everyone's blood sugar got back to normal.

My story is not original but I want to be sure to share it, so that anyone who has struggled with sickness or tragedy, or just life in general, knows my testimony of God's faithfulness. I want everyone to know that we serve a great and mighty God who is always beside us during both the good times and the bad. He wants to be there to give you strength and, to help you through whatever you are facing. Every day is a gift, just like the sweet chocolate that made Bernadette so happy. There is a sweetness and Joy that only comes from the Lord and I want it as I start each new day! How about you? ***Are you ready to MAKE THE MOST OF EVERY DAY?***

<u>CHECKUP</u>

1. In what ways have you been working for the Lord each day?

2. Is there anything that you feel the Lord is calling you to do that will help you make the most of every day?

3. Do you feel like you have been focusing more on what is going on in your life and what *you* want to do?

4. Where have you seen the Lord opened opportunities to shine His light to those around you?

5. What ways can you use your situation to help others make the most of each day they have?

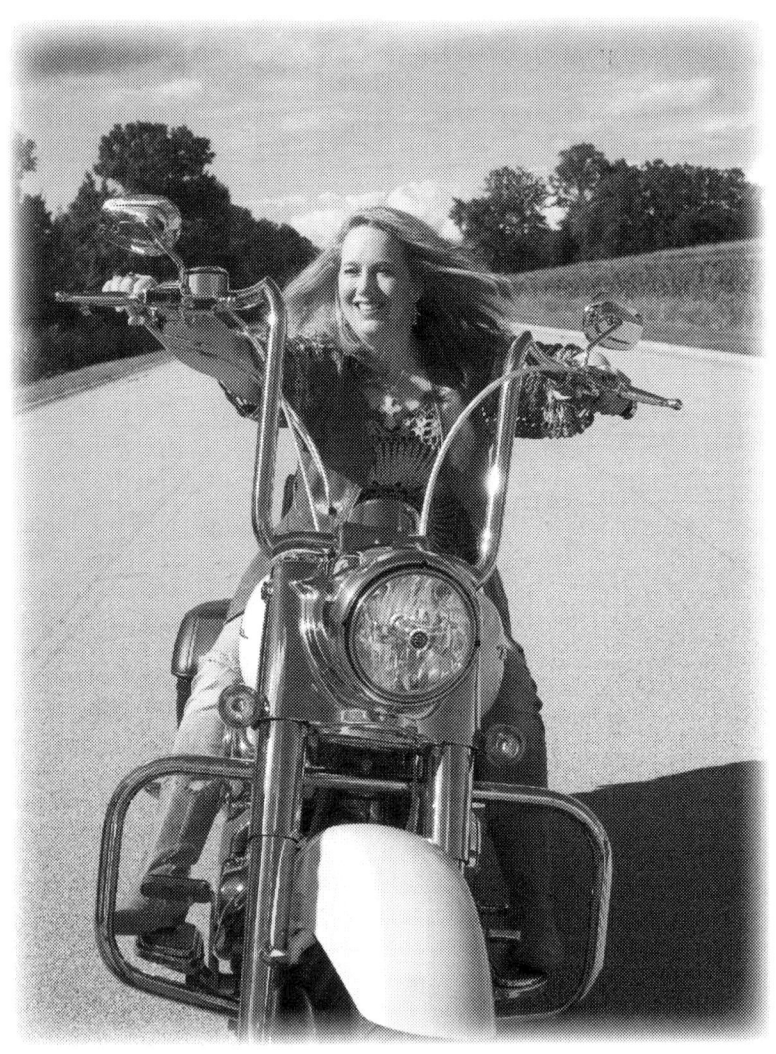

Be fearless as you follow where the Lord is leading you!

SCRIPT THREE

IDENTIFY WHAT IS REALLY IMPORTANT!

Let your light so shine before men, that they may see your good works, and glorify your Father which is in heaven. Matthew 5:16 (NIV)

There are so many things that are going on in our lives today that it is easy for us to overlook what is important and of eternal significance. Especially when facing a major life event or health crisis that calls for all of our attention. I know that I struggled to find a focus for my attention until I felt the Lord urging me to question "What really matters?" At that moment I recognized the need in my life to IDENTIFY WHAT IS REALLY IMPORTANT!

That may not sound like some great epiphany, but anyone who has struggled through a major life event really needs to follow the message of this prescription. It can remind them to gain perspective and not be overwhelmed by their circumstances.

As I look back over my life I can see so many times that I allowed myself to get sucked into something that I was doing and allowed it to take precedence over things in my life that should have been my top priority. The devil is the duke of distraction and can make us believe that we have to spend all of our time and energy on trivial things. We have to prioritize our lives, especially when times are tough. Once we identify what really matters, it is so much easier to focus on any opportunities to be a light, especially through our situation.

We need to look at the bigger picture to see not only what God is calling us to do, but what He is preparing us to do. He is calling us to be a light in a dark world, and there is no time more perfect than right now to Shine God's light, in spite of our circumstances, into the lives of those around us... It is so important in these troubled times to reach out and truly treasure the people around us that God has put in our lives.

My circumstances made me realize now more than ever that God gives us opportunities in every situation to shine His light and to appreciate all He has blessed us with.

I challenge you today to ask God to bring people into your life that need Him, and allow you to be a living example. I start to think of the song we use to sing in Sunday School that says "This little light of mine, I'm gonna let it shine" and that keeps me inspired to be a light to those around me every day! *I have identified what is important in my life and I definitely want to SHINE for Jesus... How about you?*

CHECKUP

1. What are there things in your life that are taking top priority?

2. Is there anything that you feel the devil is using to distract you from the plans God has for your life?

3. Is there something that you feel God is calling you to do?

4. What are some ways that you can shine your light for Christ?

5. What are the things in your life that are really important to you, your family and to God?

LET GO OF THE SMALL STUFF

Cast all your cares on him because he
cares for you. 1 Peter 5:7 (NIV)

Earlier in our prescriptions, we talked about submitting everything to the Lord so that we can experience all that He has planned for us and get through those uncertain times. Now, it is great to say you are submitting your life to Christ, but if you are not willing to hand every little thing over that is holding your thoughts and your actions captive, you will still be struggling throughout your circumstance. I know that it is hard, but we need to make an active choice to hand over ALL of our cares to God. We need to be sure that we even LET GO OF THE SMALL STUFF that can get in the way of our victory over our circumstances. What this means is that we need to totally trust God and also believe that He is going to take care of us.

I really love our scripture in 1 Peter and it is such a visual representation of what we need to do. The Lord really knows how to get our attention and the best words to use so we understand. The word cast tells us that we literally need to chuck or throw our cares and He will take care of it because He loves us. In the Psalms we see a similar scripture to 1 Peter 5:7 that says the Lord will also sustain us when we cast our cares on Him. What a comfort it is to read these promises!

> *"Cast your cares on the Lord and he will sustain you; he will never let the righteous be shaken."*
> *Psalms 55:22 (NIV)*

It is funny how even though I KNEW that I needed to do this, there were so many times that I just kept hanging on to all of those things that were stealing my time, my peace, my strength and my JOY.

I know that struggles and trials are temporary, and yet there are times I would cling to them. It can be hard to give it over to God, because we don't know what is going to happen. We can't see what He does and what we are really doing is trying to stay in control of our situation.

Control is definitely something that I had to learn to give to the Lord. At the risk of sounding like a broken record, we really do not have control of anything except our choices and how we respond to the things that happen to us. That really does relieve our pressure; we can hand all of it over to the Lord because we really can't do anything about it anyway. *I know I want to let go of the Small stuff that keeps me free from so many added burdens. How about you?*

CHECKUP

1. What are some of the things in your life that you are hanging on to?

2. Are any of those things affecting your life or your family?

3. Do you always feel like you need to be in control of your situation?

4. Can you recall a time in your life that you felt weighed down by too many burdens?

5. Can you list a few changes that you will make in your life to let go of the "SMALL" stuff?

SCRIPT FIVE

ENCOURAGE OTHERS

*Therefore encourage one another and build each other up,
just as in fact you are doing. 1 Thessalonians 5:11 (NIV)*

The best decision I made throughout my recovery was to follow the
Lord's example to **E**NCOURAGE OTHERS! I cannot even tell you
what a difference it made in my own outlook, and what a purpose
it gave to my life. When you go through something that literally
takes away everything that you were able to do before, it is so easy
to allow the devil to convince you that you will never be the same,
that you will never be able to do what you once did for yourself and
certainly would not be able to work for the Lord. I was very active
in ministry both at church, as well as in my own ministry to women
called Girls Just Want to Love God. The Lord had opened doors for
me to be a light to so many over the years.

As I struggled to get through the surgery and was working to
just function on my own, I was afraid that my days of ministering

to others was over. How could I be an encouragement to someone else when I was struggling to even feed myself? Those self-centered thoughts were devastating. I had no idea that the Lord would show me He still had so much for me to do and it wouldn't matter where I was in the recovery process.

As I look back throughout my recovery, I am amazed and even smile at how, day after day, circumstance after circumstance and through one person after another, the Lord renewed my call to be an encourager to those around me.

One particularly hard day comes to my mind as the first in a long line of reminders of what the Lord had called me to do. Maybe it was in spite of, or possibly because of, my circumstances that the Lord chose to use me in the way that He did.

As I had finished a very hard day of therapy, I was very teary and feeling somewhat overwhelmed. Everything made me cry; you know, the ugly kind of crying with those big crocodile tears. The worst part about it was that I had no clue why I was feeling the way I did. Sure, things were hard, but what made today any different? I realized that again, I needed to go to the Master Physician.

As I laid there in my bed for the night, I asked the Lord to renew His purpose in my life and to help me to focus on others and stop focusing on myself and my circumstances. I knew that I was miserable because I was having tunnel vision and the only thing I was looking at was myself. Once again, right then and there, the Lord touched my heart. I decided to stop thinking about what I was unable to do and change my circumstances. I was going to do things to help and encourage others that were there in the hospital unit with me.

I made a plan and had my husband get some cards printed with an image that I had used for my ministry page on Facebook some time back. The image had Proverbs 17:22 (NIV) on it... ***"A Happy Heart is good medicine"***. The other side had the following message:

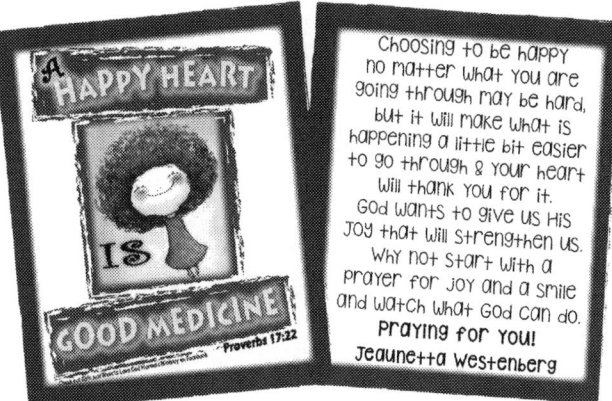

Choosing to be happy no matter what you are going through may be hard, but it will make what is happening a little bit easier to go through and your heart will thank you for it. God wants to give us His JOY that will strengthen us. Why not start with a prayer for joy and a smile and watch what God can do. Praying for you! Jeaunetta Westenberg

I would have my family take me to different rooms to deliver a card, and even pray for other patients in the unit. As soon as I was able to wheel myself around, I would make my own deliveries. I cannot tell you how doing that changed my outlook over my entire situation and blessed my life. I was meaning to encourage others, and yet I was the one who was encouraged the most. The Lord knows exactly what we need, when we really need it. When you ask the Lord for something, you really need to expect something big. I could have sat around and stayed miserable in my own tears, but I knew that the Lord was faithful to His promises, and He still had work for me to do. I want you to also know that NO matter what you are going through, God has a job for you to do that will encourage others and bless you in the process. **BE READY, BE EXPECTANT AND BE WILLING TO ENCOURAGE SOMEONE ELSE!** It can change your life… It did mine!

CHECKUP

1. How do you make yourself feel better when going through a difficult time?

2. Write down a time in your life that you were able to turn your thoughts toward someone else even when you had a need?

3. What do you think helps you to remember to focus on others?

4. Can you list a few people that may need some encouragement right now?

5. What are some things that you can do to encourage others?

One of my favorite little songs from childhood really helped me as I was experiencing sadness over my situation...

Let the Sun Shine in by Stuart Hamblen really did make a difference for me. Of course, I changed it just a little to better suit my needs because, I needed the SON more than the sun. We all do!

> *So, let the SON shine in, face life with a grin*
> *Smilers never lose and frowners never win*
> *So, let the SON shine in, face life with a grin*
> *Open up your heart and let the SON shine in*

You may be going through something hard right now. It might even seem to you like an impossible situation, but this prescription can help. It won't cure or deliver you from all that is going on, but it will sure make a difference as you go through it.

Take a look at this prescription once more and know that the best thing to do in every situation is to **SMILE!**

S: *SUBMIT YOURSELF TO THE LORD*
M: MAKE THE MOST OF EVERY DAY
I: IDENTIFY WHAT IS IMPORTANT
L: LET GO OF THE SMALL STUFF
E: ENCOURAGE OTHERS

A ROOM WITH A VIEW

What wonderful insights the Lord gave me as I took each step toward recovery. Some things were rather obvious while others had quite a learning curve, but all of them helped me get through one of the hardest times in my life.

It was very important for me to keep notes on what I was going through during some of the most difficult times. Looking back on some of the things I had written down about my long stay in the hospital was interesting. I was most perplexed by one of the notes that I had written the day prior to my surgery. It was right there in my little sparkle notebook... only 4 small words that read "A room with a view." As I read it now, and you may have guessed the same, it seemed I was hoping to have a room in the hospital that had a big window, allowing me to see the sunshine, people, nature and other beautiful things. But, it turns out, it was nothing like that... As I continued to read some of the other cryptic writings in my journal, I soon discovered that I was not talking about what I could see, I was talking about what I would need to focus on. I had other words listed on the page such as GOOD, HAPPY, PEACEFUL, STRONG,

COURAGOUS and PATIENT. It didn't take me long to realize that I didn't want a room with a view for me; I wanted a room that others could view Jesus in.

I sure wish I would have been able to put those things together and tell myself that when I was first in the hospital. It would have reminded me from the beginning how important my attitude and my focus would be, but I truly believe the lessons I learned, and the struggles I endured, will become blessings to others as I am faithful to share my story. Oh, how I long to continue to have a room with a view! God has a wonderful plan and can work through my circumstances and I can testify to that and so much more.

During my hospital stay, I wanted so badly to keep my chin up and to be a "Whatsoever Gal" that I made up some "rules" for my caregivers. As they came into my room to see me, they were only "allowed" to enter if they did one of the following:

- Tell me a joke
- Sing me a song
- Wear a bow tie
- Bring a treat (Chocolate was preferred)
- Do a dance or exercise move
- Give hugs

It was awesome to see the joy it not only brought to me, but to anyone who participated. My birthday that year was wonderful as my Doctors all arrived with fun bow ties and treats. They all told jokes, sang cute songs and even performed a few token dance and exercise moves. It was just what the Doctor ordered!

I am continually grateful for all the Lord has done and for those who have been a part of my life and my recovery. I am delighted at the small rays of "Sonshine" He allows to shine on me just when I need them.

Sometimes God even works through the simple things. While visiting the Doctor the other day, I flinched as she touched my back with the cold stethoscope to listen to my lungs. Almost immediately, I began to smile and even chuckle a little as she continued to check. That cold stethoscope reminded me that I am alive, that God has brought me through so much, and He continues to be with me no matter what comes next. Sure, I still struggle with my health, a pituitary tumor and a neuromuscular disease that limit my physical abilities and my endurance, but I am smiling and I can have a room with a view, because of Jesus. I want people to see Him through me and to recognize that even in the thick of the battle, we can celebrate victory. We can focus on the good in our situation and strive to be a "Whatsoever Gal/Guy", claiming Philippians 4:8 (KJV)…

> *Finally, brethren, whatsoever things are true, whatsoever things are honest, whatsoever things are just, whatsoever things are pure, whatsoever things are lovely, whatsoever things are of good report; if there be any virtue, and if there be any praise, think on these things.* **Philippians 4:8 (KJV)**

I know what it feels like to be out of control, to feel vulnerable, to be in pain and to experience hopelessness. I have experienced fear and anxiety that kept me from many blessings, but I am so thankful for the foundation of Joy that the Lord gave to me. Thank you for allowing me to share how the Lord was there to calm and guide me, even when I was overwhelmed with an anxious heart. In my story, I changed the way I was seeing my circumstances, and I was able to go from panic to peace. In your story, you can give it all to the Lord and let Him do the same for you. Let us say it out loud, over and over again…

DON'T Panic, It's Only _____! (Brain Surgery for me but insert whatever you are dealing with here)

DON'T PANIC GUIDES

I believe the Lord leads us through situations and allows us to learn things that will be a blessing to others. It is my utmost desire to allow the Lord to use my circumstances for His glory. I have written down a few short "How to" guides that just might help you or someone you know as they are navigating some stormy seas.

Please use the guides to help yourself and others. They are filled with things that I wish I knew before my surgery.

I also believe that if my caregivers, friends and family had something like this, it would have helped them as they were assisting me in my recovery.

DON'T PANIC GUIDE TO PRAYING FOR YOURSELF

It is so important to go to the Lord when we are in need, but it can be hard to even find the words to say when you are going through a difficult time. Here is a guide with verses that can help direct your thoughts and prayers for yourself.

Pray Continually: 1 Thessalonians 5:16-18
Pray Directly: Psalm 145:18
Pray Fervently: Hebrews 4:16
Pray Expectantly: Mark 11:24
Pray Thankfully: Colossians 3:17

DON'T PANIC GUIDE TO HELPING YOURSELF

Anytime you are going through a tough time, you really need to give yourself some grace, as you navigate the rocky waters of your circumstance. Healing takes time and you need to take care of yourself.

- **Don't try to "Act Brave or Strong"...** We certainly need to stay positive, but it is OK to let people know that you need some support.
- **It is OK to be STILL...** Sometimes the best thing for yourself and your circumstances, is to just lay low and allow the Lord to bring others into your life to help you get through the tough days.
- **Talk to people...** Share what you are going through and tell people what you need. This is the best way to communicate and be your best advocate.
- **Plan for the future...** No matter what you are going through, you will have a much better outlook if you have plans for the future. Look ahead and at first, plan small things like a dinner out. This will give you things to look forward to.

DON'T PANIC GUIDE TO PRAYING FOR OTHERS

Faithful prayer warriors are vital to those who are battling a difficult situation. Keep these scriptures in your heart and mind as you accept the call to flood the throne of grace for someone in need. If someone needs prayer, there is no better time than now to lift them up to the Lord. I read most verses in NIV translations.

Pray Personally: James 5:14-16
Pray Faithfully: Ephesians 6:18
Pray Fervently: Mathew 21:22
Pray Expectantly: 1 John 5:14
Pray Thankfully: Colossians 4:2
Pray with Power: Psalm 107 28:30

DON'T PANIC GUIDE TO HELPING OTHERS

When you are going through a tough time, there is no greater help than the love and support of a faithful friend.

- **Don't try to "FIX" everything...** Sometimes, your companionship is all that is needed. Listen, support and pray. It is ok to NOT have all the answers.
- **Don't say "If you need something, just give me a call..."** When your friend is ill, or overwhelmed with something in their life, they will not think to call or may not have the energy, but may still be in need.
- **Call your friend just to chat...** When someone is going through a difficult time, sometimes that is ALL they ever hear about and they may LOVE to just talk about everyday things like the weather.
- **Don't forget about your friend...** If your friend is going through a long-term illness or grief, it can get harder as time goes on. Everyone is there to help and comfort in the beginning, which is wonderful, but the loneliest times can come months later. Be there for your friend and keep checking in.

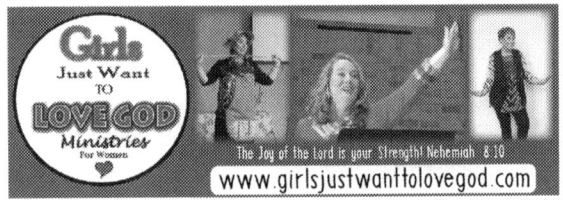

Girls Just Want to Love God Ministry for Women

Girls Just want to Love God is a non-denominational Ministry for Women. Jeaunetta started this "Friendship and Encouragement" ministry to share love, encourage, pray for others and present the Gospel message in a fun and upbeat way. It is the mission of Girl's Ministries and Jeaunetta's greatest desire for you to know the JOY that only God can give.

If you are in need of a friendly ear, a prayer warrior, or just a little encouragement; send us a note on Facebook or at girlsjustwanttolovegod.com on our contact us page. We would love to pray for you and to also share how God changes lives when we come to Him together.

The goal of Girl's Ministries is to encourage women to be all that God has called them to be.

We do this through exciting and fun programs and conferences that always point to Jesus. Our programs are interactive and one-of-a-kind and meant to delight and entertain with a message that will help us in our daily walk with Christ.

Jeaunetta speaks from the heart and would love to share all that God has done in her life with your group. If you are looking at a speaker for a Mother/Daughter banquet, Women's Retreat, Sunday Service, Christmas Tea or Community Outreach program, visit the website for contact information.

All programs are humorous, inspiring and equipping each woman to be all that God has called her to be!

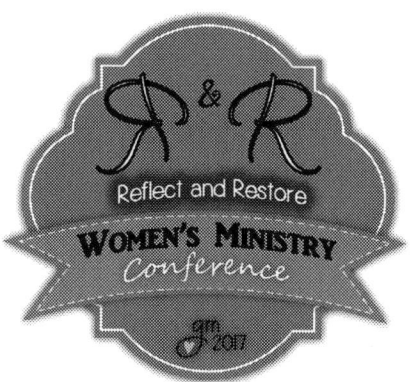

Check out our newest conference title at Girl's Ministries! The R&R Conference will help us to Reflect on who "we think" we are, and discover that, no matter how we view ourselves, or what we have been through, God can Restore us to all He has created us to be. His restoration powers are miraculous!

You can also invite Jeaunetta to come and share the program **"Don't Panic, it's Only Brain Surgery!"** at your next event. Like this book, it is an inspirational and uplifting message of victory that points directly to God; the source of her strength and resilience.

Go to our website to preview some of the program titles to get an idea for your next conference or event. There are many wonderful themes to choose from or let us know your topic and we will create a custom message that is just right for your event. All programs come with a press kit that includes digital files for bulletin inserts, posters, invitation cards and press releases.